PocketGuide to Brain Injury, Cognitive, and Neurobehavioral Rehabilitation

PocketGuide to Brain Injury, Cognitive, and Neurobehavioral Rehabilitation

Thomas J. Guilmette, Ph.D., ABPP
Director of Neuropsychology
Rhode Island Hospital & Southern New England Rehabilitation Center
Clinical Assistant Professor
Brown University School of Medicine
Providence, RI
Consultant, Southeast Rehabilitation Center at Charlton Memorial Hospital
Fall River, MA

THOMSON
DELMAR LEARNING™

Australia Canada Mexico Singapore Spain United Kingdom United States

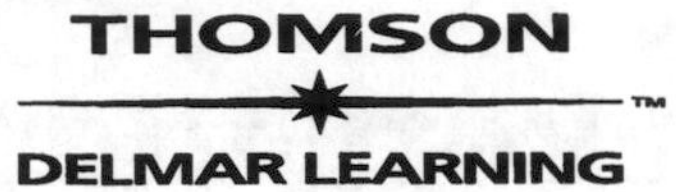

Pocket Guide to Brain Injury, Cognitive, and Neurobehavioral Rehabilitation
by Thomas J. Guilmette

Printed in the United States of America

For more information contact
Delmar Learning,
Executive Woods,
5 Maxwell Drive,
Clifton Park, NY 12065-2919
Or find us on the World Wide Web at
http://www.delmarlearning.com

Library of Congress
Cataloging-in-Publication Data
Guilmette, Thomas J.
Pocket guide to brain injury, cognitive, and neurobehavioral rehabilitation/Guilmette
p. cm.
Includes bibilographical
references and index.

1. Brain damage—Patients—Rehabilitation—Handbooks, manuals, etc. 2. Cognition disorders—Patients—Rehabilitation—Handbooks, manuals, etc. 3. Neurobehavioral disorders—Patients—Rehabilitation—Handbooks, manuals, etc. I. Title.
[DNLM: 1. Brain Injuries—complications—handbooks. 2. Brain Injuries—psychology—handbooks. 3. Brain Injuries—rehabilitation—handbooks. 4. Cognition disorders—rehabilitation—handbooks. 5. Behavioral—physiology. WL 39 G962p 1997]
RC387.5.G85 1997
616.8'046—DC21
DNLM/DLC 97-22897
for Library of Congress CIP
ISBN-13: 978-1-5659-3833-5
ISBN-10: 1-5659-3833-X

NOTICE TO THE READER

Publisher does not warrant or guarantee any of the products described herein or perform any independent analysis in connection with any of the product information contained herein. Publisher does not assume, and expressly disclaims, any obligation to obtain and include information other than that provided to it by the manufacturer.

The reader is expressly warned to consider and adopt all safety precautions that might be indicated by the activities herein and to avoid all potential hazards. By following the instructions contained herein, the reader willingly assumes all risks in connection with such instructions.

The Publisher makes no representation or warranties of any kind, including but not limited to, the warranties of fitness for particular purpose or merchantability, nor are any such representations implied with respect to the material set forth herein, and the publisher takes no responsibility with respect to such material. The publisher shall not be liable for any special, consequential, or exemplary damages resulting, in whole or part, from the readers' use of, or reliance upon, this material.

ABBREVIATED CONTENTS: ENTRIES BY DISORDERS

Foreword

We all struggle with the many difficult, if not at times bizarre, neurobehavioral/cognitive problems that present in a range of clinical settings and practices. It is a challenge to keep straight all the complex terms (e.g., anosognosia, aprosody) and categories (e.g., types of aphasia). You repeatedly see these and similar terms in medical records and neuropsychiatric assessments, but it is hard to remember what they are or what they mean. Knowledge of the brain and its functions has increased substantially, and lectures, rounds, or articles in this area excite and yet, more than occasionally, overwhelm at the same time. If only there was a quick reference to refresh or inform you at a given moment.

More difficult than knowing terms and recognizing the phenomena is what to do about them. Developing a major neurocognitive rehabilitation plan with a team is hard work. More important, you need to know what to do during your everyday therapy or other clinical encounters. How do you address memory, attention, awareness, orientation, and similar difficulties? Again, if only there was a quick guide!

This book addresses both of these needs by providing a concise, authoritative, and clear guide to neurocognitive phenomena and interventions to address them. I have worked closely with Dr. Guilmette in several different rehabilitation settings. I have always been struck by his superb ability to diagnose and to identify and explain in a clear understandable way the central features of cases. However, as I frequently tell others, "talk to Dr. Guilmette because he will not only tell you what the problem is, he will suggest good interventions to help the person deal with the problem and/or how you can get around the problem to maximize your work." This book provides the definitions and intervention strategies that all helping professionals can use in addressing the problems of those with neurobehavioral and cognitive difficulties. I like the alphabetical bullet format that gets you where you want to be quickly and easily. There is a lot to be gleaned in an easy manner. I enjoyed reading the book. I enjoyed even more knowing that I had an effective and efficient way to get back to material anytime I needed it. This book should be kept in a handy place. It is a superb and rich resource.

Duane S. Bishop, M.D.
Providence, Rhode Island

Preface

Persons with traumatic brain injury (TBI) and other neurologic disorders with neurobehavioral consequences pose particular challenges to rehabilitation professionals. The rehabilitation of cognitive and neurobehavioral deficits is labor intensive and often frustrating due to the ambiguous nature of the field. Although there are many references available that offer both theoretical and clinical approaches to the remediation of neurobehavioral deficits, this PocketGuide was written to provide rehabilitation professionals with concise and easily referenced cognitive and behavioral rehabilitation interventions for patients with brain injury and related neurologic disorders. It also includes definitions of terms that clinicians may encounter frequently when working with this patient population.

The treatment suggestions contained in this work are meant to be pragmatic, focused, and easily implemented. They are intended to provide a starting point from which clinicians can modify and expand interventions as necessary. In order to accomplish this, decisions were made to exclude the theoretical constructs underlying a procedure and whatever disagreements may exist in the field regarding the efficacy of a specific intervention. The choice of whether to include or exclude any treatment approach was based on the author's clinical experience and understanding of the available scientific literature. Undoubtedly, some worthy treatment interventions were inadvertently excluded and some less efficacious ones included. The reader should understand that no specific treatment suggestion necessarily applies to all patients. For any errors of omission or commission, the author bears full responsibility.

It is important to recognize that this PocketGuide is designed for clinicians with some background in brain function and rehabilitation. As such, it is intended for clinicians who evaluate and treat persons with neurologic disorders that affect cognitive and behavioral functioning. It is appropriate for the new clinician and students as well as more experienced professionals. Clinicians in the fields of occupational therapy, physical therapy, speech-language pathology, therapeutic recreation, rehabilitation nursing, vocational rehabilitation, rehabilitation psychology and psychiatry, social work, and neuropsychology may find some benefit in this book.

The reader will notice some overlap among the interventions listed. This is inevitable given that cognitive abilities do not exist in isolation of each other and that the brain functions as an integrated unit. The overlap also exists because certain themes in cognitive rehabilitation are important and need to be integrated in most interventions: consistency of treatment and increasing patients' awareness of their deficits, for example.

With few exceptions, there are no endorsements of specific cognitive rehabilitation manuals, computer programs, or workbooks. This PocketGuide was not intended to survey the commercial products available in this clinical area. Rather, the treatment suggestions are meant to be easily applied with minimal resources. However, this most certainly is not meant to imply that treatments should be applied in a "cookbook" fashion. Each patient is unique and needs to be approached as such. Treatment suggestions should *never* be applied without a proper assessment and understanding of the patient on the part of individual clinicians and of the treatment team. The suggested interventions should never be a substitute for clinical judgment.

The PocketGuide also contains a number of terms describing neuroanatomical structures that are relevant to cognitive and behavioral functioning as well as descriptions of neuropathological processes and behavioral/psychological issues often encountered in the rehabilitation of persons with brain injury. Again, some important terms may have been inadvertently excluded, although every effort was made to include the concepts most relevant to practitioners working in neurorehabilitation. There are also names of some specific tests and evaluation procedures that are frequently used but which some rehabilitation professionals may not be completely familiar with. Although there are hundreds of tests that assess the cognitive functioning of persons with brain injury, an effort was made to provide descriptions of only a very limited sample of the more common procedures.

Some terms and interventions are followed by references. These citations refer to works that were relied on to describe the term or intervention or that the reader can refer to for more information. Some references were relied upon more than others, particularly, *Neuropsychological Assessment* (Lezak, 1995), *Clinical Neurology for Psychiatrists* (Kaufman, 1995), *Principles of Behavioral Neurology* (Mesulam, 1985), and *Introduction to Cognitive Rehabilitation: Theory & Practice* (Sohlber & Mateer, 1989).

Some interventions and treatment suggestions cannot be referenced but have been developed informally over time by dedicated clinicians, some of whom I have had the privilege of working with in over 10 years in neurorehabilitation. I have benefited greatly from their creativity, their experience, and their ideas, and I am in their debt. It is also important to acknowledge the patients and families who have allowed us to struggle with them in developing treatment procedures for some of the devastating cognitive and behavioral problems resulting from brain injury. We have learned much from our patients and I thank them for their trust and honesty. Last, a loving thank you to my family, to my parents, Ruth and Rene, and to my wife, Mary, and our children, Andrew and Jay, who have supported me unconditionally and allowed me the opportunity to pursue (at times selfishly) my own interests and ideas.

How to Use This PocketGuide

This PocketGuide is organized like a glossary, with terms and treatment suggestions listed in alphabetical order. Each main entry is printed in bold type and may define a type of disorder seen in neurorehabilitation (e.g., Traumatic Brain Injury, Cerebrovascular Accident, or Subarachnoid Hemorrhage), a neuroanatomical structure (e.g., Thalamus), a description of a cognitive or behavioral ability associated with brain function (e.g., Attention or Memory), or the name of an assessment procedure used in neurorehabilitation (e.g., Glasgow Coma Scale). Terms that describe a specific cognitive ability are usually followed by specific treatment suggestions and interventions. Any term that is cross-referenced is underlined. Within each heading there may be subcategories that provide additional information about the topic and in some cases references are provided for the reader's further interest.

Some of the main entries that may be of interest to the reader include the following:

Abulia
Adjustment (to disability or deficits)
Agitation
Aphasia
Arousal
Attention
Awareness
Behavioral Management
Cerebrovascular Accident
Cognitive Rehabilitation
Coma
Constructional Ability
Dementia
Executive Functions

Frontal Lobes
Memory
Neglect
Orientation
Perceptual Functioning
Problem Solving
Social Skills Training
Traumatic Brain Injury

To my wife, Mary, and our two sons, Andrew and Jay

Abducens Nerve. Cranial Nerve VI; originates from the Pons; innervates the lateral rectus muscle of the eye; important for lateral eye movement and conjugate gaze along with Cranial Nerves III and IV; impairment causes inward deviation of the eyeball and Diplopia when looking toward the temple; affected by Brain Stem lesions including trauma, Hemorrhages, Tumors, etc.

Abstract Thinking. The ability to think in useful generalizations; to infer from single instances; to understand concepts and to be capable of using reason and logic to solve problems; associated with Problem Solving and Conceptual Thinking; the absence of abstract capabilities results in Concrete Thinking.

- Not related to any one specific brain area although the Frontal Lobes play some role in the ability to form abstract concepts
- Problems in this domain usually result from diffuse or widespread brain damage
- Higher levels of education are usually associated with better functioning in this area
- Aging tends to adversely affect this ability
- Abstract thinking can be measured through proverb interpretation, by asking how two concepts or objects are alike, such as a leg and an arm (this is an example of the type of item found on the Similarities subtest of the Wechsler Adult Intelligence Scale-Revised), or other tests such as the Wisconsin Card Sorting Test and the Category Test
- Abstract thinking deficits are difficult to rehabilitate; see treatment of Problem Solving deficits for suggestions

Abulia. An inability to initiate or complete activities due to decreased or absent drive; has been associated with Basal Ganglia, Limbic System, and Frontal Lobe brain injuries; the disorder is not due to Depression or other Mood Disorders; can have a significant impact on a patient's ability to care for self independently, maintain a household, find and maintain employment, and structure free time (the latter is a very common complaint among family members of persons who have sustained TBI); this disorder is difficult to treat effectively. See also Executive Functions.

Treatment of Abulia

- Rule out Depression or other Mood disorders (treat if present)
- Rule out other cognitive deficits that could account for inability to initiate or complete tasks such as Apraxia, deficits with Memory and Attention, or impairments of reasoning and Problem Solving
- Attempt to engage patient in familiar and intrinsically interesting activities, such as hobbies enjoyed prior to the injury
- Establish written daily schedule:
  - This should be established with the patient's input
  - The daily activities listed should include the times they are to be initiated
  - The activities should be concrete, objective, and measurable (i.e., write "dust the living room furniture" rather than "clean the house")
  - Begin with small goals or tasks to be accomplished and limit the number to one or two initially
  - List each and every task that is to be performed rather than combining them into one item (i.e., every step for ADLs may need to be listed rather than simply "perform AM routine")
  - Each task that is accomplished should then be crossed off the list
  - Goals and activities need to be updated frequently with the patient's input
  - An alarm watch may alert patient to refer to the schedule
  - Post the schedule in many locations in the patient's home or hospital room
  - Instruct family and friends to reinforce and encourage patient to keep to the schedule
  - Attempt to have the patient make a verbal commitment to accomplish the tasks on the schedule
  - Use praise and reward for completing tasks

  - As patient demonstrates ability to accomplish tasks, gradually increase their number
- If possible, make frequent but brief checks on the patient to encourage, prompt, and reinforce task accomplishments
- Do not scold or otherwise humiliate patients for inability to complete tasks; they are not lazy
- Use Behavior Management principles to increase compliance, particularly with positive reinforcement and reward; initially reinforce even close approximations to the desired behavior (i.e., praise patient for getting to the sink even if he or she failed to begin grooming activities)
- Determine if patient's activity level or initiative fluctuates during the day and incorporate that information into schedule
- Use behaviors that patient engages in more spontaneously as reinforcement to accomplish other tasks
- Educate patient about effects of injury
- Consider psychotropic medications (e.g., psychostimulants), if not medically contraindicated, to increase drive
- Give only one command or instruction at a time
- Allow patient sufficient time to respond to a request before moving on to the next task or command
- Use gentle touch to help patient initiate action
- Demonstrate the task that you wish the patient to begin; this modeling may assist the patient to begin the activity
- Use heightened inflection and Prosody in voice to "energize" patient

Acalculia. An inability to perform arithmetic calculations; it is usually associated with lesions to the left Parietal Lobe or adjacent areas; when found in connection with other conditions, it may be referred to as an Angular Gyrus Syndrome or Gerstmann's Syndrome; in children with Right Hemisphere Learning Disabilities, calculation or arithmetic abilities are frequently inferior to reading skills.

Acalculia, Spatial. An inability to perform written calculations due to incorrect number placement and an inability to keep numbers properly aligned in rows and columns; the patient is able to perform mental calculations without difficulty; this disorder is due to problems with Perceptual Functioning usually associated with Posterior Right Hemisphere lesions; performing written calculations on graph paper may help to keep numbers properly aligned.

Achievement Tests. Tests of academic skills such as reading, vocabulary, math, spelling, and so forth, usually administered at regular intervals during primary and junior high school; examples of group administered Achievement Tests include the Metropolitan Achievement Test and the Iowa Test of Basic Skills; examples of individually administered Achievement Tests are the Wechsler Individual Achievement Test and the Wide Range Achievement Test; these types of tests are not measures of aptitude or Intelligence; they assess the academic skills the child or adult has already learned; it is helpful to obtain these test results in a school-age child or young adult to make an estimation of premorbid functioning.

Achromatopsia. A complete or partial loss of color vision in a quadrant, hemifield, or the whole visual field; usually associated with occipitoparietal damage.

Acoustic Nerve. Cranial Nerve VIII; originates from the Pons; composed of two divisions: the cochlear division controls hearing and the vestibular division controls equilibrium, body position, and orientation to space; damage to the cochlear nerve can cause Tinnitus and deafness; damage to the vestibular nerve can cause Vertigo and Nystagmus; these disorders can be caused by Traumatic Brain Injury.

Acoustic Neuroma. A benign tumor of the Acoustic Nerve; does not result in cognitive deficits.

Acquired Immunodeficiency Disorder (AIDS). Results from infection of the human immunodeficiency virus type 1 (HIV-1), which creates opportunistic infections, Tumors, and cerebrovascular disease; an estimated 40–70%

of patients will develop clinical neurologic abnormalities; up to 25% of HIV-1 patients may develop a Dementia as their initial symptom of AIDS and an additional 15% may develop Dementia with other symptoms; the "AIDS dementia complex" now known more formally as the "HIV-1-associated cognitive/motor complex" may involve the following signs and symptoms:

- Problems with Concentration and Memory
- Decreased Mental Speed and slowed thinking
- Slowed and clumsy motor movements
- Gait incoordination and Ataxia
- Apathy, social withdrawal, and reduced spontaneity
- Incontinence
- Myoclonus

Stern, R. A., Perkins, D. O., & Evans, D. L. (1995). Neuropsychiatric manifestations of HIV-1 infection and AIDS. In F. Bloom & D. Kupfer (Eds.), *Psychopharmacology: The fourth generation of progress* (pp. 1545–1558). New York: Raven Press, Ltd.

Adjustment (to disability or deficits). A psychological or emotional reaction to an injury, disability, or deficit.

- The most common reactions are Depression, Anxiety, changes in self-esteem, sense of loss, withdrawal or social isolation, anger, and denial or minimizing deficits (these latter two reactions should not be confused with an organic denial or Anosognosia, which are the direct result of brain trauma and are not psychologically based)
- Personality changes can also occur following brain injury which can be the direct result of organic factors or brain damage
- Adjustment problems can affect participation in rehabilitation, a willingness to use compensatory strategies, and relationships with others
- Family Functioning can also be affected by adjustment problems that need to be addressed
- Many adjustment problems arise during the postacute rehabilitation period

- For families of survivors of head injuries, the second 6 months of the first posttraumatic year is often when psychological and emotional issues first become prominent

Treatment of Adjustment Problems

- A person's adjustment to his or her disability will be based on several factors including the type of injury, age, other psychosocial stressors, Personality variables, and so forth, all of which will need to be considered in how the team interacts with the patient
- Patients may interact and exhibit different emotions with different therapists depending on what the therapist is asking them to do (some evidence suggests that among elderly rehabilitation patients, more emotional distress is directed at nurses and that the fewest emotional problems are noted during physical therapy)
- Give patients the opportunity to discuss their feelings and reactions about their problems but do not pry or assume that they must be having a particular experience because that is how you would feel
- Encourage the patients to be as productive as possible in spite of their disabilities (people need to feel needed and useful)
- Encourage the patient's independence and pride in his or her accomplishments
- Try to help patients focus on what they can do, not on what they can't do
- Remind patients of their progress; acknowledging even small gains is important
- Don't minimize the patient's feelings by making comments like "Oh, don't feel like that" or "You shouldn't feel like that"
- Don't suggest that you know how the patient must feel (avoid comments such as "I know exactly how you feel")
- Encourage patients to compare their progress from some point after their injury or illness (e.g., in the last few weeks or months) and not compare their current functioning with their premorbid status

- Do NOT take away a patient's hope for at least some minimal and continued improvement or adaptation to his or her disability
- Offer support groups for patients and their families
- Educate patients and families about the nature of their illness, trauma, and disability
- Refer the patient for psychotherapy or counseling to a mental health professional (psychologist, psychiatrist, social worker, rehabilitation counselor) who has experience in working with this population
- Refer to a psychiatrist if there is a question of whether medications, such as antidepressants, might be helpful

Caplan, B., & Shechter, J. (1987). Denial and depression in disabling illness. In B. Caplan (Ed.), *Rehabilitation psychology desk reference* (pp. 133–170). Rockville, MD: Aspen Publishers, Inc.

Guilmette, T. J., Snow, M. G., Grace, J., & Giuliano, M. S. (1992). Emotional dysfunction in a geriatric population: Staff observations and patients' reports. *Archives of Physical Medicine and Rehabilitation, 73,* 587–593.

Affect. An outward and observable expression of emotion; it refers to the fluctuating change in emotions; examples include sadness, elation, and anger; affect may be broad or full (normal) or may be restricted in some manner.

Examples of Abnormal Affect from the Diagnostic and Statistical Manual of Mental Disorders (4th Edition)

- *Blunted:* A significant reduction in the intensity of emotional expression
- *Flat:* Absence or near absence of any signs of emotions
- *Restricted or constricted:* Mild reduction in the range and intensity of emotional expression
- *Inappropriate:* Discordance between emotional expression and the content of speech or ideation (e.g., laughing while talking about a sad or tragic event)
- *Labile:* Abnormal variability in affect with repeated, rapid, and abrupt shifts in emotional expression

- The term Pseudobulbar Affect is also used to describe Lability although there is some question whether the two terms represent the same condition
- With Lability, there is an assumption that the affect reflects the emotional state of the individual (e.g., when the person cries it is because of sadness) but with Pseudobulbar Affect the Lability may not necessarily be due to a change in emotions (there is a great deal of overlap in how these two terms are used)
- Lability can also be referred to as pathological laughing and crying.

Affective Disorders. Refers to disorders of Mood, such as Depression.

Aging Effects. The effects of aging on brain and cognitive functions can be quite variable and must be taken into account in the assessment and rehabilitation plans of elderly persons who have sustained brain trauma; obtaining a good premorbid history of the individual's functional abilities (i.e., ability to manage household tasks such as finances, medications, etc.) and cognitive skills, particularly short term Memory, is important in determining appropriate goals for rehabilitation; the use of age-appropriate norms in testing speech and cognitive functions is essential; a summary of clinical issues related to aging is listed below:

- Many of the healthy elderly retain normal levels of cognitive functioning even through the eighth decade (there is a great deal of variability in the cognitive abilities of older persons, which makes it difficult to provide global statements about functioning in this area)
- Advancing age increases the likelihood of developing many neuropathological disorders including Dementia, Cerebrovascular Accidents, brain Tumors, cardiovascular insufficiency, and multi-system organ failures that can adversely affect cognitive functioning
- There is a decline in brain volume likely due to neuronal shrinkage and selective cell loss (this may result in cortical

Atrophy and increased ventricular size although it is not necessarily related to Dementia or a significant loss of cognitive abilities)

- Although not true in all cases, advancing age can be associated with poorer outcome following brain trauma
- Sensory and motor loss are common
  - Hearing is decreased in up to 70% of persons over 70
  - Decreased visual acuity, scanning efficiency, and light-dark adaptation
  - Odor sensitivity is reduced
  - Decreased motor speed, coordination, and strength
  - Accommodations for these problems within the rehabilitation setting will be necessary
- Sleep patterns also change with age (see also Sleep Disorders)
  - Nighttime sleep is shorter and more fragmented, which may result in more daytime naps
  - Sleep onset and awakening tend to be earlier
  - Sleep patterns and need for rest should be incorporated into the rehabilitation schedule of elderly patients
- Decreased Mental Speed or information processing is one of the most common cognitive effects of aging (elderly patients may require more time to process new information and respond to new environments)
- Other common cognitive changes that can accompany normal aging include:
  - Decreased sustained and divided Attention
  - Less efficient and slower rates of learning new information (the elderly may require more practice, time, and rehearsal to absorb new material)
  - Poor spontaneous recall of information (for both remote and newly learned information) that can be significantly aided by cueing and recognition (see Memory)
  - Problems reproducing (copying) complex geometric designs but accurate productions of simpler ones
  - Decreased ability to solve new or novel problems (increased Concrete Thinking) which may affect a person's ability to adapt to new situations or environments

- Cognitive functions that are most resistant to aging include: vocabulary and verbal skills in general; reading; remote or long term Memory; arithmetic problem solving; retention of newly learned information if tested in a recognition format; simple Attention and Concentration abilities
- Cognitive changes tend to be less pronounced in the elderly with higher levels of education and who are generally healthier
- Depression in the elderly can result in significant cognitive deficits (known as Pseudodementia) which are reversible with treatment; psychiatric referral and consultation would be important for treatment of this disorder
- In persons with a pre-existing mild Dementia, a neurologic insult such as a Cerebrovascular Accident or head injury can result in substantially greater deficits than if the condition occurred in an individual without Dementia
- A change in environments, such as hospitalization, can exacerbate pre-existing cognitive problems (individuals often function much better in their own homes or in familiar environments than in institutional settings)
- During acute rehabilitation try to keep patients on a daily schedule that matches their own at home with regard to naps (if they took one), time to get up in the morning, and sequence for performing activities of daily living
- Try to keep rehabilitation activities functional and meaningful for patients as they may not always understand the purpose of the activities or techniques being taught
- Allow the elderly patient more time to process information and practice new techniques
- Ensure that the patient can hear adequately, even if he or she has a hearing aid

Aggression. Violent behavior, usually directed at or toward an object or person; there is significant overlap with Agitation and irritability although aggression may be more purposeful and goal directed; see Agitation for treatment recommendations.

Agitation. Not a well-defined concept; often used interchangeably with restlessness, Aggression, Impulsivity, Disinhibition; usually refers to a heightened state of activity with evidence of irritability, behavioral dyscontrol, and decreased cooperation with therapeutic activities; agitation is often different during acute recovery (i.e., within weeks or months of the injury when the patient is still confused or in Posttraumatic Amnesia) than during the postacute period (i.e., months to years postinsult); see Agitation in Postacute Rehabilitation below for further distinctions.

- Brooke, Questad, Patterson, & Bashak (1992) defined agitation and restlessness as two different types of behavior
  - *Agitation* was defined as episodic, requiring restraint or medication to prevent damage to persons or property, significantly interfering with patient care, and may be motoric (hitting, agitated pacing, dislodging of catheters, throwing objects, combativeness) or verbal (belligerence, swearing, threatening, making denigrating remarks to others)
  - *Restlessness* was defined as continuous, not interfering significantly with safety, and that it may require some action on the part of the staff but it does not interfere significantly with patient care
- Corrigan and Bogner (1994) defined agitation as composed of Aggression (violence, anger, self-abusiveness, resistant to care) and other nondirected or restless behavior; Disinhibition (impulsivity, distractibility, wandering, pulling at tubes, pacing) and Lability (repetitive behaviors, mood changes, rapid, loud, or excessive talking); see Agitated Behavior Scale
- The Rancho Los Amigos Cognitive Scale describes Level IV as "confused-agitated," when a patient is in a heightened state of activity, responds primarily to his or her own internal confusion; may be aggressive, bizarre, euphoric, or hostile

- Studies have revealed that approximately one-third to one-half of brain injured patients will exhibit periods of agitation and/or restlessness during their recovery

Factors That May Increase Agitation in Acute Rehabilitation

- Confusion and disorientation, especially to time and place, are highly associated with agitation (usually prominent during acute rehabilitation while the patient is in Posttraumatic Amnesia but is less common during postacute rehabilitation)
- Intoxication at the time of trauma
- Agitation in the acute care hospital
- Extent of diffuse brain injury (the greater the extent of neurologic deficits, the greater the likelihood of agitation)
- Male gender
- Shorter periods of Coma
- Medical comorbidity (especially cardiovascular disease and hypertension)
- Medication interactions and side effects
- Pain and physical discomfort of the patient
- Metabolic encephalopathies and Delirium
- Overstimulation
- Restraints and other devices that limit the movement of the patient
- NOT associated with Traumatic Brain Injury alone; other neurologic disorders such as CVA, Hypoxia, etc. can also result in agitation

Treatment of Agitation in Acute Rehabilitation

- May require multiple and varied approaches; must individualize to the patient
- Pharmacologic intervention may be necessary although it may
  - Produce sedation
  - Accentuate confusion and impede cognitive recovery
  - Produce paradoxical effects of intensifying aggressive behavior

- Physical restraints may also be necessary but may
  - Potentiate agitation by increasing feelings of powerlessness and lack of control
  - Result in pain which can increase confusion and agitation
  - Create greater disability (and in rare cases, death) if not used properly
- Behavioral and environmental interventions (which require close coordination among team members and a systematic approach to patient care; are labor intensive; can create stress among staff; and require continual training and education) are listed below:
  - Do not expect the patient to act "normal" (remember that the patient is unable to control his or her behavior and that the world has become a very confusing and frightening place)
  - Rule out an underlying Aphasia that may interfere with communication and further increase agitation
  - Do not continue with an activity that is increasing the agitation
  - Select staff that are most comfortable with this population
  - Rule out metabolic or medication side effects that may be increasing agitation
  - Expected the unexpected
  - Develop a consistent plan about how to react to the patient and ensure that all staff are aware of it
  - Confused patients are most comfortable with people they know—make liberal use of family in treatment to calm, reassure, and orient the patient
  - Give patients space to "walk off" restlessness but try to keep them in same general area for familiarity
  - Make patient's room as familiar as possible by placing pictures of family, home, etc. in plain view; put objects in the room that the patient may find some comfort in such as a favorite blanket, pajamas, etc.
  - Orienting information, such as month, year, and place should be plainly visible and easy to read

- Provide the patient with pictures of therapists and their names as a way to begin orienting the patient to his or her surroundings
- Avoid restraints whenever possible
- Control stimulation such as lights, noise, general activity level, visitors, etc. (keep lights dimmed, reduce noise level both inside and outside the patient's room, control traffic in the corridors)
- Try to keep the patient's daily schedule the same each day and post it in his or her room
- Use short, but frequent sessions
- Control fatigue level and monitor endurance as these factors can contribute to agitation
- Use familiar or overlearned functional activites to engage the patient; attempt to have the patient participate in hobbies or activites that he or she found interesting premorbidly
- The fewer words to communicate the better; try to use sentences of 10 words or less in length
- Use words and vocabulary that the patient understands
- Try to keep activities meaningful and consistent with the patient's psychosocial history
- Reorient the patient at the beginning and end of each treatment session
- Stay calm if the patient is escalating
- Reassure patient with a calm soothing voice (patients are often frightened because they do not understand what has happened to them)
- Use distraction if patient is Perseverating or if agitation is increasing
- Staff and family should use the same words or phrases to describe to the patient why he or she is in the hospital (e.g., "You were in a car accident and hit your head"); this minimizes confusion and potentially conflicting messages to the patient; consistency in this area also begins to increase insight and Awareness of injury

- Reinforce and reward (socially) calm and appropriate behavior
- Do not scold the patient for agitation or inappropriate behavior
- Try to ignore inappropriate behaviors, unless they compromise the patient's safety
- Be sensitive to patient's physical comfort (pain and other noxious stimuli can be hyperirritating to patients, especially in some Frontal Lobe syndromes, and can increase agitation)
- Monitor agitation through behavioral monitoring and attempt to identify Antecedents that may escalate Aggression or agitation
- Avoid room changes
- Gradually increase demands and independence of the patient as he or she can tolerate
- Staff who have the best relationship with the patient, regardless of discipline, should help calm the patient when escalating
- Educate family and visitors about how to interact with the patient (e.g., limit stimulation, do not argue with patient, etc.)
- See Rancho Los Amigos Cognitive Scale and Behavior Management

Agitation in Postacute Rehabilitation

- Agitation in the postacute recovery period is usually less frequent and less intense than during acute recovery (irritability and short-temper, however, are frequent sequelae to Traumatic Brain Injury and to other forms of brain damage)
- When agitation occurs after the acute recovery period, it is usually in response to a specific environmental, social, or psychological stressor (e.g., being denied a request or as a reaction to a perceived insult; during acute rehabilitation, agitation can occur when the patient is alone and with minimal, if any, stimulation or Antecedents)

- Advantages to treating agitation during postacute rehabilitation are the improved cognitive status of the patient (e.g., better Memory, Attention, reasoning, lack of confusion in all but the most severe brain injuries), the ability of the patient to participate in therapies, and the ability to identify specific precipitating events that lead to agitated behavior
- Agitation and excessive irritability can cause significant interpersonal and family problems that lead to social isolation of the patient; it is a major cause of impaired vocational functioning
- Agitation and Aggression can result from lesions to the Hypothalamus, Temporal Lobe Epilepsy, Frontal Lobe syndromes, frontotemporal insults, multifocal and metabolic disorders, and psychiatric disorders such as Delusions, Depression, and Mania

Treatment of Agitation in Postacute Rehabilitation

- Rule out reversible etiologies or contributing factors such as Seizures, metabolic disorders, and psychiatric conditions
- A thorough neuropsychological assessment is warranted to determine cognitively what types of interventions, feedback, and strategies the patient can tolerate
- Assess Mood, Anxiety, and other psychological states
- A major treatment approach is with Behavior Management techniques and other environmental and psychosocial interventions
- Developing a program to decrease agitation or Aggression requires (1) observing the patient for instances of Aggression; (2) defining the problem in concrete, behavioral terms; (3) defining and selecting the target behavior to modify; (4) establishing a baseline; (5) graphing the frequency of the behavior; (6) selecting a treatment intervention; (7) evaluating the efficacy of the intervention
- Provide praise and other reinforcement for positive behavioral responses
  - Describe inappropriate and appropriate behaviors (in specific and concrete terms)

- Review continually the rationale for the intervention
- Increase Awareness of how the patient's behavior affects others, family functioning, ability to hold a job, make and keep friendships, etc.
- Teach and practice appropriate behavioral responses
- Give patient frequent feedback about progress
- Consider techniques such as Behavior Contracts, Extinction or time out, and Token Economies
- Consider Social Skills Training
- Teach patient to anticipate problems and to think about what responses would be most appropriate in a given situation
- Treat in a group format when available (this allows for feedback from others and the opportunity to practice new behaviors)
- Deal with Adjustment to disability and other psychological isssues such as Depression and Anxiety through individual or group psychotherapy
- Include in treatment the patient's family and others that interact frequently with the patient and train them also in how to intervene at times of agitation or Aggression
- Consider altering the patient's environment if specific stressors or precipitating events consistently lead to increased agitation and if other interventions have been unsuccessful

- Consider pharmacologic approaches via consultation with a psychiatrist, neurologist, or Neuropsychiatrist

Berrol, S. (1988). Risks of restraints in head injury. *Archives of Physical Medicine and Rehabilitation, 69,* 537–538.

Bishop, D. S., & Pet, R. (1995). Psychobehavioral problems other than depression in stroke. *Topics in Stroke Rehabilitation, 2,* 56–68.

Brooke, M. M., Questad, K. A., Patterson, D. R., & Bashak, K. J. (1992). Agitation and restlessness after closed head injury: A prospective study of 100 consecutive admissions. *Archives of Physical Medicine and Rehabilitation, 73,* 320–323.

Corrigan, J. D., & Bogner, J. A. (1994). Factor structure of the Agitated Behavior Scale. *Journal of Clinical and Experimental Neuropsychology, 16,* 386–392.

Galski, T., Palasz, J., Bruno, R. L., & Walker, J. E. (1994). Predicting physical and verbal aggression on a brain trauma unit. *Archives of Physical Medicine and Rehabilitation, 75*, 380–383.

Lewis, F., Burke, W. H., & Carrillo, R. (1987). Model for rehabilitation of head injured adults in the post acute setting. *Journal of Applied Rehabilitation Counseling, 18*, 39–45.

Saver, J. L., Salloway, S. P., Devinsky, O., & Bear, D. M. (1996). Neuropsychiatry of aggression. In B. S. Fogel, R. B. Schiffer, & S. M. Rao (Eds.), *Neuropsychiatry* (pp. 523–548). Baltimore, MD: Williams & Wilkins.

Agitated Behavior Scale. A 14-item rating scale designed to reliably and objectively rate a patient's Agitation during acute rehabilitation; the scale seems to tap three basic constructs: Disinhibition, Aggression, and Lability; the scale can be used monitor a patient's progress or to evaluate the efficacy of an intervention.

Corrigan, J. D., & Bogner, J. A. (1994). Factor structure of the Agitated Behavior Scale. *Journal of Clinical and Experimental Neuropsychology, 16*, 386–392.

Agnosia. The inability to recognize or know the meaning of stimuli, when presented, in spite of intact intelligence, alertness, and ability to communicate; this deficit usually occurs in one sensory modality at a time, such as visual or auditory, but leaves recognition in the other sensory modalities intact; descriptions of the various agnosias listed below are summarized from Mesulam, M. M. (1985). *Principles of behavioral neurology*. Philadelphia: F. A. Davis Company.

- **Auditory agnosia.** The inability to interpret or recognize auditory stimuli in spite of intact hearing; auditory agnosia is divided into two types:
  - **Verbal auditory agnosia**, also known as pure word deafness, results in a disturbance of spoken language comprehension and repetition with normal verbal output and intact reading and writing (Wernicke's Aphasia [as described under Aphasia] differs in that verbal output and reading are usually impaired with a disturbance of auditory comprehension); the neuropathology may

involve the area around Heschl's Gyrus in the left hemisphere or the middle portions of the first temporal gyrus bilaterally

- **Nonverbal auditory agnosia** is the inability to recognize nonlanguage sounds such as a doorbell, the telephone ringing, a car driving by, etc.; this usually results from right temporal damage

- **Finger agnosia.** The inability to name fingers or point to, name, or recognize a finger that has been touched by the examiner; not due to Aphasia or sensory loss; one of the four elements of Gerstmann's Syndrome; associated with dominant (left) hemisphere lesions usually in the Parietal Lobe or in the area of the parietal-occipital junction
- **Visual agnosia.** The inability to recognize an object that is presented visually in spite of intact naming and perception; the patient will usually be able to describe or draw the object that he or she is seeing, but will be unable to recognize it or know what it is; if the patient feels or palpates the object, then recognition will likely occur; visual agnosia is often accompanied by Achromatopsia; this disorder is rare; it may result from bilateral lesions in the occipitotemporal visual areas

Agrammatism. The lack of use of proper function words, such as articles and prepositions, and appropriate endings to words such as plurals, tenses, and possessives; this may be seen in written and/or spoken language.

Agraphia. The inability to write; usually occurs with other language or Aphasia symptoms, including the inability to read (Alexia), although in rare cases writing may be intact but reading is impaired (Alexia without Agraphia); when agraphia occurs due to a central language disorder then the lesion is frequently in the area of the left temporoparietal region; there may be a partial or a complete inability to write letters or words; agraphia is one of the four elements of Gerstmann's Syndrome; in some cases an inability to write due to poor handwriting and physical problems, rather than an underlying language disorder, is also referred to as agraphia if the writing sample is illegible.

Akinesia. A lack of or altered physical movements.

Akinetic Mutism. A lack of responsiveness to the environment both verbally and motorically; the patient may appear alert but is generally immobile and does not speak or respond to stimuli; bilateral lesions to the Anterior portions of the Cingulate Gyrus will cause this disorder (usually from strokes in the territories of the Anterior Cerebral Artery or the Anterior Communicating Artery); see also Locked-in Syndrome.

Alcohol Effects. Alcohol (ethanol, abbreviated ETOH) is a central nervous system depressant and is considered to be a neurotoxin.

- The effects of alcohol on brain function can be quite variable and are dependent upon a number of factors, including:
  - Length of time the person has been drinking
  - Age at which the individual began abusing alcohol
  - Amount of alcohol consumed
  - Family history of alcoholism
  - Biological vulnerability to alcohol
  - The person's overall health and nutritional status
  - How long the individual has been abstinent from alcohol (if that is the case)
- Assessing and treating alcohol use in rehabilitation is important because alcohol may affect brain/cognitive functions which in turn can adversely impact a person's response to rehabilitation
- There is also a significant relationship between alcohol use and Traumatic Brain Injury, as studies have revealed that up to 50% of persons who sustain a brain injury have a significant blood alcohol level (i.e., intoxicated) at the time of trauma
- The next two sections will review the effects of alcohol on brain function with and without brain injuries

Alcohol Effects in Persons Without Brain Injuries

- Chronic alcohol use substantially increases the risk of multiple organ disease and may affect the liver, gastrointestinal tract, immune and endocrine systems, and the central nervous system
- Alcoholics are at high risk for head injuries (from driving while intoxicated or from falls that may result in multiple mild head injuries) and nutritional disorders, as alcohol is high in calories but has no nutritional value (see <u>Korsakoff's Syndrome</u>)
- Brain <u>Atrophy</u>, abnormal EEG findings, and reduced regional cerebral blood flow have been reported in chronic alcoholics
- Withdrawal from alcohol can result in <u>Seizures</u> and delirium tremens (i.e., tremulousness, <u>Hallucinations</u>, confusion, <u>Agitation</u>)
- Chronic alcohol use can result in difficulties (of varying degrees) in short-term <u>Memory</u>, <u>Perceptual Functioning</u>, motor speed, <u>Abstract Thinking</u>, and <u>Executive Functions</u>
- Language functions and remote or long-term <u>Memory</u> remains relatively unaffected in alcoholics
- Deficits in cognitive functions vary greatly among chronic alcohol abusers
- Serious and profound <u>Memory</u> deficits are not a typical feature of alcoholism unless the individual develops a more prominent <u>Korsakoff's Syndrome</u>
- During detoxification (usually within the first 2 weeks of abstinence), alcoholics may exhibit more severe deficits in a wide range of cognitive functions than they would routinely when still drinking
- Abstinence from alcohol often leads to improvement in cognitive functions, particularly for individuals under age 40, although some deficits may persist; improvement may occur within weeks to months of cessation of drinking
- Younger alcoholics may also be at risk for other substance abuse disorders

Goldman, M. S. (1983). Cognitive impairment in chronic alcoholics: Some cause for optimism. *American Psychologist, 37,* 1045–1054.

Lezak, M. D. (1995). *Neuropsychological assessment* (3rd ed.). New York: Oxford University Press.

Parsons, O. A. (1994). Determinants of cognitive deficits in alcoholics: The search continues. *The Clinical Neuropsychologist, 8,* 39–58.

Alcohol Effects in Persons with Brain Injuries

- A significant blood alcohol level at the time of head trauma has been associated with lower levels of Consciousness, lower cognitive status at discharge, adverse long-term effects on Memory, longer duration of Coma, and longer periods of Agitation
- Although some studies have reported that alcohol use may decline following brain injury, the incidence of alcohol use in TBI survivors has been estimated at around 40%, with 20% of those individuals described as moderate to heavy drinkers
- Alcohol is known to lower the Seizure threshold which places individuals with TBI at even higher risk for Seizures
- The use of alcohol and other illicit drugs *following* brain injury has been associated with increased Seizures, worsened cognitive deficits, poor social functioning, increased likelihood of subsequent head injuries, greater behavioral deficits, and negative interactions with prescribed medications
- In the postacute period, alcohol use has been linked to criminal behavior and vocational impairments (see Vocational Rehabilitation)

Kreutzer, J. S., Doherty, B. A., Harris, J. A., & Zasler, N. D. (1990). Alcohol use among persons with traumatic brain injury. *Journal of Head Trauma Rehabilitation, 5,* 9–20.

Kreutzer, J. S., Marwitz, J. H., & Wehman, P. H. (1991). Substance abuse assessment and treatment in vocational rehabilitation for persons with brain injury. *Journal of Head Trauma Rehabilitation, 6,* 12–23.

Sparadeo, F. R. (1993). Substance use: A critical training issue for staff in brain injury rehabilitation. In D. Durgin, N. Schmidt, &

L. Fryer (Eds.), *Staff development and clinical intervention in brain injury rehabilitation* (pp. 189–205). Gaithersburg, MD: Aspen Publishers, Inc.

Solomon, D., & Sparadeo, F. R. (1992). Effects of substance use on persons with tramautic brain injury. *NeuroRehabilitation, 2,* 16–26.

Assessment and Treatment of Alcohol Use in Persons with Brain Injury

- The effects of brain injury on cognitive functioning, particularly with Insight and self-awareness, Memory, Impulsivity, Disinhibition, and Problem Solving, must be considered when working with this population
- Including a substance abuse professional, particularly one with experience in working with TBI survivors, on the treatment team will be necessary to effectively manage and treat patients currently abusing or at high risk for alcohol use
- Assessment of alcohol risk should include:
  - Past history of alcohol use
  - Cravings or urges for alcohol or other substances
  - A family history of alcohol or substance abuse
  - Family members or friends currently with an alcohol or substance abuse problem
  - The presence of alcohol "triggers" or stimuli in the environment that prompts/reminds the individual to drink
  - Level of family and psychosocial support available
  - Family's prior and current view of the patient's alcohol or substance abuse
  - Presence of additional psychosocial stressors (e.g., marital, financial)
  - See Alcohol Screening for a brief listing of some commonly used screening instruments
- The overall treatment goal is the prevention of future alcohol use; abstinence is the objective
- Individuals at low risk for alcohol use (e.g., negative history of abuse, no cravings or urges, intact and healthy support systems, negative family history of alcoholism)

can usually be treated with education (that matches their cognitive abilities) about the risks of alcohol use, encouraging family support and awareness of alcohol problems, helping patients recognize "high risk" situations, such as being in places where alcohol is readily available, and helping them problem solve about what to do in those circumstances

- All treating therapists must reinforce the issues outlined here and be consistent in their messages about why it is important to abstain from using alcohol
- A current user or a person at high risk for future use requires a more integrated and intensive treatment approach, including:
  - More comprehensive assessment of drinking history and family functioning
  - A matching of the patient's specific needs with the appropriate interventions
  - An educational program that increases awareness of the substance abuse problem and the necessity for change
  - Skill building in how to cope with the urge to drink and how to handle situations in which alcohol is present

Sparadeo, F. R. (1993). Substance use: A critical training issue for staff in brain injury rehabilitation. In D. Durgin, N. Schmidt, & L. Fryer (Eds.), *Staff development and clinical intervention in brain injury rehabilitation* (pp. 189–205). Gaithersburg, MD: Aspen Publishers Inc.

Sparadeo, F. R., Strauss, D., & Kapsalis, K. B. (1992). Substance abuse, brain injury, and family functioning. *NeuroRehabilitation, 2,* 65–73.

Alcohol Screening. There is no definitive or "gold standard" alcohol screening instrument although many screening tools exist; given the high incidence of alcohol and substance abuse in individuals with brain injury, many authors have advocated routine screening of all persons with TBI; alcohol screening instruments, however, should not replace a careful clinical interview by a mental health professional if alcohol abuse is suspected; examples of alcohol screening instruments are listed below:

- Brief Michigan Alcohol Screening Test (Porkony et al., 1972)
- Quantity Frequency Variability Index (Cahalan & Cisin, 1968a, 1968b)
- Substance Abuse Subtle Screening Inventory (Miller, 1985)
- Addiction Severity Index (McClellan et al., 1980)
- CAGE questions (Ewing, 1984); a rating of 2 or more on the 4 CAGE questions (see below) is considered significant for alcohol problems; these questions can be quickly and easily administered as part of routine screening for all rehabilitation patients.
  - Have you ever tried to Cut down on your drinking?
  - Do you ever get Annoyed or angry when people criticize your drinking?
  - Do you ever feel Guilty about your drinking?
  - Do you ever have an Eye opener (i.e., a drink in the morning to relieve a hangover or withdrawal symptoms)?

Cahalan, D., & Cisin, I. (1968a). American drinking practices: Summary of findings from a national probability sample: I. Extent of drinking by population subgroups. *Quarterly Journal of Studies on Alcohol, 29,* 130–151.

Cahalan, D., & Cisin, I. (1968b). American drinking practices: Summary of findings from a national probability sample: II. Measurement of massed versus spaced drinking. *Quarterly Journal of Studies on Alcohol, 29,* 642–656.

Ewing, J. (1984). Detecting alcoholism: The CAGE questionnaire. *Journal of the American Medical Association, 252,* 1905–1907.

Fuller, M. G., Fishman, E., Taylor, C. A., & Wood, R. B. (1994). Screening patients with traumatic brain injuries for substance abuse. *Journal of Neuropsychiatry and Clinical Neurosciences, 6,* 143–146.

Miller, G. A. (1985). *The Substance Abuse Subtle Screening Inventory Manual.* Spencer, IN: Spencer Evening World.

McClellan, A. T., Luborsky, L., Woody, G. E., et al. (1980). An improved diagnostic evaluation instrument for substance abuse patients: The Addiction Severity Index. *Journal of Nervous and Mental Diseases, 168*, 26–33.

Porkony, A. D., Miller, B. A., & Kaplan, H. B. (1972). The Brief MAST: A shortened version of the Michigan Alcohol Screening Test. *American Journal of Psychiatry, 129*, 342–345.

Alexia. The inability to read; frequently accompanies other language disorders in Aphasia; the patient may be partially or fully unable to read words or single letters; see also Dyslexia.

Alexia, Central. An inability to read or write (Agraphia); described by Mesulam (1985) as "a return to illiteracy"; associated with dominant (left) hemisphere Parietal Lobe lesions.

Mesulam, M. M. (1985). *Principles of behavioral neurology*. Philadelphia, PA: F. A. Davis Company.

Alexia Without Agraphia. An inability to read but with preserved ability to write; the individual cannot read words but can recognize words spelled aloud and write them when asked; a right homonomous Hemianopsia is often present; lesions in the dominant hemisphere Occipital Lobe and in the splenium (i.e., Posterior portion) of the Corpus Callosum are usually responsible for this syndrome.

Alien Hand Syndrome. A relatively uncommon syndrome in which a patient's arm and hand, usually on the left, will explore the environment in a disinhibited or semipurposeful manner; patients will often report no ability to control the limb, or in extreme cases may deny that the hand is theirs; a lesion in the Corpus Callosum has been associated with this disorder.

Alzheimer's Disease. Known also as Dementia of the Alzheimer's Type (DAT); it is the most common cause of dementia, accounting for at least half of all dementias; it is a progressive disease process that results in a gradual but insidious decline in a person's cognitive, behavioral, and adaptive functioning; listed below are additional factors regarding this disease.

- The history and course of Alzheimer's disease are important to understand because many patients in rehabilitation centers are elderly and age is the single biggest risk factor for this disorder
- The underlying neuropathology is the development of high numbers of neurofibrillary tangles (tangles of fine fibers found in cell bodies) and senile plaques (extracellular by-products of neuronal degeneration)
- Although there are many theories, there is no known cause
- Some studies have linked Alzheimer's disease to a history of head trauma although others have not
- Confirmed diagnosis can only be made by autopsy; there is no definitive test for Alzheimer's disease, including a CT scan or Magnetic Resonance Imaging
- The presence of Alzheimer's disease does not exclude a person from having other neurologic disorders such as Parkinson's Disease or strokes
- The most common early symptom is declining short-term Memory, which the patient may or may not be aware of (later in the disease process, there is no awareness of deficits)
- A Memory problem alone does not necessarily indicate that the patient has Alzheimer's disease
- Other early symptoms may include a deterioration in speech and communication, particularly naming, verbal fluency, spelling, comprehension, and the meaningfulness of speech
- As the disease progresses, patients will exhibit deficits with Perceptual Functioning, reasoning, Problem Solving, Abstract Thinking, and Apraxia; patients eventually become confused and unaware of their surroundings, are unable to care for themselves and become completely dependent on others

- During the early to middle stages of the disease, long-term or remote Memory remains intact relative to the short-term Memory deficit; this may mislead families into believing that the patient's Memory is intact because he or she can recall events that happened decades ago (although events that happened very recently are not retained)
- Behavioral and emotional changes are also common, including Depression, Apathy, irritability, restlessness, and Agitation
- In the early to middle stages of the disorder, patients can become more confused by being away from home, such as in a hospital
- Studies have revealed a range of 1½ to 15 years for the duration of the disorder
- Questioning the patient, and more important the family, about the patient's short-term or recent Memory prior to his or her hospitalization may provide some clues about a preexisting Dementia (Memory problems alone, however, are not sufficient for a diagnosis of Dementia); if Memory problems are reported, then ascertaining whether they have progressed or gotten worse over the recent past may provide some evidence of whether this may be a deteriorating condition (please see the Dementia entry for more information and caveats about making a diagnosis)
- If Alzheimer's disease is suspected, then a thorough neurologic evaluation is suggested to rule out a reversible Dementia
- A neuropsychological evaluation is recommended to determine if cognitive problems exceed normal aging and to assess whether the patient's cognitive profile is consistent with Alzheimer's disease or other neurocognitive disorders
- A diagnosis of Alzheimer's disease does not preclude participation in rehabilitation although goals may need to be modified to accommodate some of the patient's limitations; in some patients the disease proceeds slowly, so

they may have relatively long periods of stable functioning to participate in and benefit from rehabilitative treatment

- The rehabilitation team should not assume that a patient with a probable diagnosis of Alzheimer's disease is incompetent or cognitively incapable of making decisions (careful assessment of each patient is necessary to determine the severity of cognitive impairments and his or her relative strengths and weaknesses)
- Family and caregiver education about home management and methods of interacting with the patient will be crucial (see Dementia entry for specific details); referral to local Alzheimer's disease support groups and other supportive/advocacy groups may assist the family to cope with the disease

Treatment Suggestions for Alzheimer's Disease

- Complete cognitive assessment by neuropsychology, speech/language therapy, and occupational therapy
- If Memory is significantly impaired (the most common finding in Alzheimer's disease), then the patient may have to keep a Memory Log to keep track of important information (see Memory entry for more specific suggestions), presuming that language functions are intact enough to allow for reading and writing
- Patients with severe short-term Memory disorders can still learn new techniques through Procedural Learning; this is the learning of new skills or motor programs through consistent and massed practice
- If the patient exhibits Apraxia, then hand-on-hand techniques may be necessary to assist with motor tasks and programs
- Place large Orientation signs in plain view of the patient if disoriented
- Keep language concrete and as succinct as possible but do not talk "down" or in a patronizing way to the patient
- Control the level of stimulation for restlessness or Agitation
- Keep interventions and methods of communicating with the patient consistent among treating therapists

- Try to engage the patient in activities or tasks that are intrinsically interesting and meaningful to him or her
- Strongly encourage family participation in treatment sessions unless it is upsetting to the patient
- Give patient choices when possible (i.e., between two treatment activities or which task he or she would like to do first)
- Gently correct patients for misidentification of people or things in their environment (e.g., believing a therapist is a relative or the hospital is the factory where they used to work); however, do not continue to correct patients if they become upset or irritable
- Use recent pictures of family members, enjoyable events, the patient's home, etc., to assist with reorientation
- See specific entries for management of disorders of Attention, Memory, Problem Solving, Orientation, Aphasia, Agitation, and Dementia

Home Management Suggestions for Alzheimer's Disease

- Patients are often more independent in a familiar environment, such as their own home, than in an unfamiliar environment, such as a hospital (home evaluations may be important to more accurately assess the patient's functional abilities and need for supervision)
- Home modifications need to be continually reassessed given that Alzheimer's disease is a progressive disease that gradually worsens with time
- Neuropsychological assessment will be helpful to document the course and progression of the patient's cognitive deficits and to assist with safety and Competence issues
- The primary goal is to keep the patient as independent as possible
- The type and amount of supervision needed will depend on the patient's level of confusion, restlessness, and Disinhibition; for example, some persons with Alzheimer's disease can exhibit Apathy and Abulia, which decreases

the likelihood that they will engage in dangerous activities if left unattended for brief periods of time; decisions in this area need to be made on an individual basis

- Try to keep the person on a routine and keep the day as structured as possible (e.g., meals at about the same time, consistent time to go to bed and get up in the morning, consistent ADL routine, etc.)
- Write the patient's daily schedule on a piece of paper in large print and post in a conspicuous place or places
- Keep Orientation aids, such as clocks, calendars, etc., in plain view and refer the patient to these consistently; make sure they are easy to read
- Create a family picture album with recent pictures of family and friends; label each picture with the name and age of the person and how he or she is related to the patient
- Put a sign on cabinets and drawers listing their most important contents (e.g., glasses, knives and forks, plates, etc.)
- Keep items that the patient uses frequently in the same place and label the area clearly
- Avoid and reduce clutter; remove unnecessary items from the tops of counters, from drawers, etc.
- Control stimulation in the home; avoid chaotic situations, large parties, loud noises, or many people visiting simultaneously
- If the patient is severely confused, then all dangerous items, such as medications, cleaning solvents, power tools, etc. should be removed or locked securely away; keep car keys out of sight; remove stove or oven knobs so that the patient would be unable to operate the appliance
- Turn down thermostat on the hot water heater so that the patient will not be in danger of burning him- or herself
- Additional materials and information can be obtained through the Alzheimer's Disease and Related Disorders Association, 919 North Michigan Avenue, Suite 1000, Chicago, IL, 60611, telephone: 800-272-3900.

Amnesia. A partial or total loss of Memory; can be caused by many conditions including, but not limited to, Traumatic

Brain Injury, Anoxia, Infarcts, brain Tumors, Herpes Simplex Encephalitis, Subarachnoid Hemorrhages, Dementia, Seizures, medication effects, and Korsakoff's Syndrome; amnesia may occur as a relatively isolated deficit, with other cognitive and intellectual functions remaining relatively intact; the most severe amnesic syndromes occur with bilateral damage to the Limbic System, particularly to the Hippocampus and/or the Thalamus; see also Transient Global Amnesia, Posttraumatic Amnesia, Retrograde Amnesia, Anterograde Amnesia, and Memory.

Amygdala. Part of the Limbic System; a Subcortical Structure within each Temporal Lobe in close proximity to the Hippocampus; involved with protective drive states, Affect, and emotional responses; isolated damage to the amygdala may or may not produce cognitive or Memory deficits although its proximity to the Hippocampus suggests some association with Memory; it may be important in establishing affective or emotional associations to events; humans with amygdalas excised tend to show little affect and spontaneity; see Kluver-Bucy Syndrome.

Aneurysm. A thin-walled, balloon-shaped dilation of a blood vessel; they tend to occur at the bifurcation and branches of arteries; within the Cerebral Circulation system aneurysms are most common (>90%) in the Circle of Willis, particularly within the area of the Anterior Communicating Artery.

- Autopsies have revealed the presence of aneurysms in 4%–17% of cases
- The peak incidence of aneurysms is between 35 and 65 years of age
- Aneurysms are usually asymptomatic until they rupture
- Angiography is the only way to demonstrate the presence of an aneurysm
- They are the leading cause of Subarachnoid Hemorrhages which can result in serious cognitive deficits and disability

- Ruptured cerebral aneurysms have a high mortality rate and complications (e.g., rebleeding, Hydrocephalus, Vasospasm) are common
- Many patients with ruptured aneurysms will require Cognitive Rehabilitation
- The size and profuseness of the bleeding resulting from a ruptured aneurysm can be graded into descriptive categories:
  - Grade I—mild bleed; alert, minimal headache, no neurologic deficit
  - Grade II—mild bleed; alert, mild to severe headache, nuchal rigidity, minimal neurologic deficit
  - Grade III—moderate bleed; drowsy or confused, nuchal rigidity, may have mild focal neurologic deficit
  - Grade IV—moderate to severe bleed; stuporous, may have mild to severe hemiparesis
  - Grade V—severe bleed; in deep Coma, decerebrate posturing

Brown, G. G., Spicer, K. B., & Malik, G. (1991). Neurobehavioral correlates of Arteriovenous Malformations and cerebral Aneurysms. In R. A. Bornstein (Ed.), *Neurobehavioral aspects of cerebrovascular disease*. New York: Oxford University Press.

Neurologic care (clinical pocket manual). (1986). Springhouse, PA: Springhouse Corporation.

Angular Gyrus Syndrome. A constellation of symptoms described by Mesalum (1985) which includes Anomia, Alexia, constructional deficits, Acalculia, Agraphia, Finger Agnosia (described under Agnosia), and left/right disorientation; these deficits may occur in the absence of generalized language comprehension impairments; lesions to the inferior Parietal Lobe may result in this syndrome.

Mesalum, M. M. (1985). *Principles of behavioral neurology*. Philadelphia, PA: F. A. Davis Company.

Anhedonia. A loss of feeling pleasure in activities that were usually pleasurable; most often associated with Depression.

Anomia. The inability to name an object on presentation or generate a specific word in spontaneous speech; also described as a problem with "word finding" or "word retreival"; the person knows what the object is (unlike a Visual Agnosia, as described under Agnosia), can describe its function and physical characteristics, but cannot give it a name; anomia is a common symptom in Aphasia but is also evident in many other neuropathological conditions in which language is relatively well preserved; lesions to many different brain structures may result in anomia; it is also associated with normal aging; see Aphasia for treatment considerations.

Anosmia. The inability to perceive smells, including the aroma of food; it is usually the result of damage to the Olfactory Nerve (Cranial Nerve I).

- Normal aging results in anosmia due to neuronal degeneration
- In younger persons, the most common causes for anosmia are Traumatic Brain Injury (the location of the Olfactory Nerve in the undersurface of the Frontal Lobes makes it particularly vulnerable to the shearing effects of TBI) and Tumors (e.g., olfactory groove Meningiomas)
- Anosmia is present in approximately 20%–30% of severe TBIs
- Studies have revealed that anosmia following TBI has been associated with chronic unemployment in a high percentage (>90%) of survivors, even for those without significant cognitive deficits, due to presumed Frontal Lobe damage
- Perceiving smells that are not present (olfactory Hallucinations) maybe a symptom of Seizures.

Costanza, R. M., & Zasler, N. D. (1992). Epidemiology and pathophysiology of olfactory and gustatory dysfunction in head trauma. *Journal of Head Trauma Rehabilitation, 7*, 5–24.

Varney, N. R., & Menefee, L. (1993) Psychosocial and executive deficits following closed head injury: Implications for orbital frontal cortex. *Journal of Head Trauma Rehabilitation, 8*, 32–44.

Anosognosia. The denial of illness or deficit due to organic or biologic factors.

- It is not the result of a psychological, emotional, or adjustment problem
- In Cerebrovascular Accidents, anosognosia is most often evident in nondominant (right) hemisphere lesions, particularly in the Parietal Lobe, and is frequently accompanied by hemiplegia, visual and somatosensory Neglect, and impaired Constructional Ability
- In moderate to severe brain injuries, lack of Awareness of deficits is a common finding and may result from Frontal Lobe or diffuse brain damage
- Anosognosia has significant treatment ramifications (see Awareness entry for further discussion and treatment recommendations)

Anoxia. A complete lack of oxygen (a reduction of oxygen is known as Hypoxia) to the brain that may be caused by cardiac or respiratory failure, near drowning, carbon monoxide poisoning, failed hanging, complications of anesthesia, chronic obstructive pulmonary disease (COPD), barbiturate overdose, or sleep apnea (see Sleep Disorders).

- The brain may use up to 20% of the body's oxygen in the resting state and has limited metabolic reserves of oxygen, thus it is highly vulnerable to the effects of a reduction or cessation in its oxygen supply (particularly vulnerable are the Hippocampus, Thalamus, Basal Ganglia, and the areas supplied by the most distal reaches of two adjoining arterial trees)
- Anoxic or hypoxic injuries can result in severe brain damage and disability, including Coma
- Memory deficits are common and may be debilitating
- Cardiac arrest has been shown to produce deficits with learning, Memory, Abstract Thinking, Attention, Concentration, Perceptual Functioning, and the capacity to plan, initiate, and carry out mental activities

- Emotional changes, most commonly, Depression, can also occur
- Comprehensive cognitive evaluation and rehabilitation may be necessary

Bass, E. (1985). Cardiopulmonary arrest. *Annals of internal medicine, 103*, 920–927.

Lezak, M. D. (1995). *Neuropsychological assessment* (3rd ed.). New York: Oxford University Press.

Roine, R. O., Kajaste, S., Kaste, M. (1993). Neuropsychological sequelae of cardiac arrest. *Journal of the American Medical Association, 269*, 237–242.

Antecedents. Events or stimuli that precede the behavior under study; in Behavior Management programs, identifying the antecedents to an undesirable behavior, such as Agitation, is an important component in developing an intervention or treatment plan; if antecedents to behavioral problems are known, then interventions can be implemented that can decrease or eliminate them which in turn may alter the unwanted behavior.

Anterior. In front of or in the forward area.

Anterior Cerebral Artery (ACA). One of the three main cerebral arteries that branches off the Circle of Willis to the medial or middle surface of the Frontal and Parietal Lobes; Aneurysms in the ACA may cause significant cognitive and/or personality alterations reflecting Frontal Lobe or Executive Function deficits; see also Anterior Communicating Artery and Cerebral Circulation.

Anterior Communicating Artery (ACoA). Within the Circle of Willis, a small artery that connects the two Anterior Cerebral Arteries; it is a very common site for Aneurysms and subsequent Subarachnoid Hemorrhages; hemorrhages that occur in the ACoA can result in a permanent Anterograde Amnesia or substantial short-term Memory impairments but most other cognitive functions remain generally intact; during the acute recovery period, the patient may be globally amnestic and exhibit evidence of Confabulation and impaired long-term Memory or Retrograde Amnesia; personality alterations can occur, such as changes with mood (Depression or euphoria) and Affect (reduced capacity to show emotion or labile/disinhibited emotional responses), as well as socially inappropriate behaviors.

Anterograde Amnesia. A loss of Memory for recent events or for activities/information that occurred after a brain trauma or insult; a deficit with short-term Memory; may result from many different neuropathological conditions, including stroke, Anoxia, Traumatic Brain Injury, and Dementia.

Anticonvulsants. A class of medications used to treat Seizures or epilepsy; the choice of anticonvulsant is based on the type of seizure and side-effect profile; persons with Traumatic Brain Injury are frequently placed on an anticonvulsant for prophylactic reasons even though they have never had a seizure; some anticonvulsants may affect cognitive abilities by increasing lethargy and fatigue which in turn can affect Attention, Concentration, Mental Speed, and Memory; anticonvulsants may have their most adverse side effects with persons who have the greatest amount of brain dysfunction.

Anton's Syndrome. A denial of blindness which can occur with Cortical Blindness; patients may insist that their vision is intact and may even describe (inaccurately) objects in their room.

Anxiety. A subjective emotional state of nervousness, worry, and apprehension; patients may also experience physiological symptoms such as sweaty palms, "butterflies" in the stomach, muscle tension, etc.

- Individuals who are somewhat "perfectionistic" are more prone to develop anxiety disorders than those who are not

- Some specific anxiety disorders include panic disorder (recurrent and unexpected panic attacks), phobias (a marked and persistent fear of a specific object or situation), agoraphobia (fear of being in a situation from which escape might be difficult or embarrassing), and obsessive-compulsive disorder (recurrent/repetitive thoughts or behaviors that interfere with daily functioning)
- Following brain insult, either from stroke or brain injury, individuals may develop anxiety disorders that were not present premorbidly or premorbid anxiety may worsen
- Anxiety problems may also accompany certain types of <u>Seizure</u> disorders
- Anxiety, uncertainty, and apprehension can interfere significantly with a patient's ability to achieve maximum benefit from rehabilitation
- The elderly, in particular, may develop a fear of falling that can interfere with transfers and ambulation
- Anxiety, especially in high levels, can interfere with such cognitive functions as <u>Attention</u> and <u>Memory</u>

Treatment for Anxiety

- Careful history taking and review of current symptoms by a mental health professional would be necessary to diagnose an anxiety disorder
- If formal treatment is required, then referral to a psychiatrist for medication use and/or a psychologist for behavioral intervention is recommended
- Rehabilitation team members can help patients deal with their anxiety in the following ways:
  - Provide verbal reassurance and comfort, but do not dismiss the patient's concerns as trivial or "silly" (although the anxiety may seem irrational, it is very real and powerful to the patient)
  - Give patients as much information as they can tolerate about their condition, their daily schedule, the rehabilitation process, etc.; anxiety tends to increase in the absence of information

- Make the patient's treatment as predictable as possible by saying, "This week we'll be working on . . ." or "Today we'll be doing . . ." (people with anxiety hate surprises)
- Because anxiety may interfere with a person's ability to concentrate and pay attention, make sure the person is listening to and understanding what you are saying
- Keep information succinct and write it down if the patient seems too anxious to absorb it all at once
- Teach relaxation procedures and techniques (e.g., deep breathing, guided imagery, deep muscle relaxation) if the patient can tolerate these interventions cognitively
- Discuss with the patient what he or she is fearful of and how you, as the therapist, can help lessen or help the patient manage those fears
- Encourage the patient to express "worst case" scenarios about the activity he/she is fearful of and try to address the probability of those occurring and how you or others would react/prevent their occurrence
- Gradually expose patients to what they are fearful of (e.g., standing, going into the community) by discussing the fearful stimuli, having patients imagine themselves in the situation, approximating the activity (do a task that is similiar), and performing the action in small increments while at the same time allowing patients to relax/compose themselves after each "small step"

Apathy. A lack of interest in the environment, people, or activities; a common symptom of Depression but may also occur as a result of a brain injury; if severe, it can significantly reduce drive and motivation (see Abulia).

Aphasia. An acquired impairment of language function that may include some or all aspects of language-dependent communication (e.g., expressive speech, receptive speech, reading or Alexia, writing or Agraphia, and repetition).

- The major aphasic syndromes that are described are based on the assumption of left hemisphere dominance (even most left handers are left hemisphere dominant for language although a minority will have language representation in the right or both hemispheres)

- Focal brain lesions in the territory of the left Middle Cerebral Artery (Frontal, Temporal, or Parietal Lobes) are usually responsible
- Vascular disorders and Dementia are the most common neuropathological conditions that cause aphasia
- Hemiparesis or hemiplegia on the right side of the body often accompany aphasia due to the proximity of the Motor and Sensory Strips to cortical language areas
- The patient's type and severity of aphasia must be considered when assessing other cognitive skills, including such rudimentary functions as Orientation (e.g., a patient with a receptive aphasia may not understand the questions asked of him or her or a patient with an expressive aphasia may not be able to name the correct month even if it is known)
- Evaluation of cognitive skills is best accomplished through the use of nonverbal assessment measures, careful observation of Problem Solving skills for functional activities, and carry-over of newly learned tasks and techniques
- Apraxia frequently accompanies aphasia and should therefore be evaluated
- Patients with aphasia and left hemisphere lesions generally may be more likely to become depressed than some other patient groups; monitoring of Mood is suggested
- The most common aphasic syndromes are listed here; it is important to note that patients may exhibit characteristics of more than one syndrome at a time

Major Syndromes of Aphasia

Broca's Aphasia. Also known as a nonfluent, expressive, frontal, or Anterior aphasia

- *Spontaneous* speech is nonfluent, agrammatical, produced as single words or short phrases, telegraphic, with absent prosody, intonation, and inflection (Aprosodia); this may cause significant frustration and distress for the patient

- *Comprehension* is relatively well preserved
- *Naming* is often but not always impaired
- *Repetition* is impaired
- *Reading* is almost always impaired
- *Writing* is almost always impaired
- *Localization* is just Anterior of the precentral gyrus in the Frontal Lobe

Wernicke's Aphasia. Also known as fluent, receptive, or Posterior aphasia

- *Spontaneous speech* is fluent with normal phrase length, prosody, intonation, and inflection, although little meaning is conveyed (content or important words are absent); there are frequent Paraphasic Errors and word substitutions; patients are frequently unaware of their errors or communication deficits
- *Comprehension* is almost always impaired
- *Naming* is almost always impaired
- *Repetition* is almost always impaired
- *Reading* is almost always impaired
- *Writing* is almost always impaired
- *Localization* is in the Posterior portion of the superior temporal gyrus

Conduction Aphasia

- *Spontaneous speech* is fluent but with Paraphasic Errors, like Wernicke's aphasia
- *Comprehension* is relatively well preserved
- *Naming* is often but not always impaired
- *Repetition* is almost always impaired; impaired repetition with relatively preserved comprehension separates it from Wernicke's aphasia (in Wernicke's aphasia, comprehension is always impaired)
- *Reading* aloud is impaired but reading comprehension is more intact
- *Writing* is almost always impaired but often to a mild degree

- *Localization* is usually in the White Matter fibers that connect Broca's and Wernicke's areas (an area known as the arcuate fasciculus)

Global Aphasia. A global language disorder resulting in impaired comprehension and expression; usually caused by large Infarcts in the left Middle Cerebral Artery producing large lesions to the Frontal, Temporal, and Parietal Lobes; patients may be mute and frequently Apraxic.

Transcortical Motor Aphasia. Similar to Broca's aphasia with the exceptions of repetition, which is intact, and reading, which is also generally well preserved; seems to involve frontal fibers in the area adjacent to Broca's area.

Transcortical Sensory Aphasia. Similar to Wernicke's aphasia but with intact repetition; damage to the area in the parietotemporal junction and the areas adjacent to Wernicke's causes this syndrome.

Suggestions for Communicating with Patients with Aphasia

- The speech therapist will be crucial in the treatment of these language disorders (specific interventions and ways of communicating with the patient will need to be individualized by the speech therapist and communicated to the treatment team)
- Keep language simple (i.e., avoid complex syntax, prepositional phrases, etc.) and utterances brief
- Do not ask open-ended questions (e.g., questions beginning with How, Why)
- Ask yes/no questions
- Speak slowly, but not loudly (the aphasic patient is not deaf)
- Allow only one person to speak at a time
- Give concrete or tangible choices to patients when asking questions
- Avoid discussing abstract concepts or using abstract language

- Give one instruction at a time
- Allow the patient time to process information before expecting a response or rephrasing a question
- Do not shift topics quickly
- Pause before changing the subject of the discussion or conversation
- Give the patient written cues (one or two words) to augment understanding of a question or when giving choices (point to the word or short phrase as it is being said)
- When using written cues, write the word(s) in upper and lower case letters as this creates a contour or shape for the word which may facilitate understanding by the Right Hemisphere
- Emphasize the use of gestures, facial expressions and voice intonation when talking with patients with aphasia as these may facilitate their understanding (this allows the brain to use nonverbal, visual cues to augment comprehension)
- Use pictures to help patients identify their needs
  - Ensure that the patient is able to understand the meaning of the pictures
  - Keep the pictures readily available at all times for the patient, staff, and family
  - Make sure that the pictures are used in a uniform and consistent manner by everyone
- If the patient is also apraxic, he or she may be unable to point, in which case give the patient a pencil or similar object to grasp and "point" with it (this allows the patient to use whole arm movements to "point" rather than small, coordinated movements, which are more difficult to produce in Apraxia)
- For patients with severe comprehension deficits, use demonstration and modeling (without any speaking) to show them how to perform activities or to teach new techniques
- All staff must be consistent in how the patient is taught new techniques, such as transfers, as there is no opportu-

nity to use language to clarify how the activity should be done or for the patient to ask questions

- Family education and counseling about the patient's language disorder and ways of communicating with him or her are crucial
- The number of visitors may need to be limited as patients may become more confused and Agitated with increased environmental auditory stimulation
- Monitor carefully the patient's frustration level, especially with a patient with a Broca's aphasia
- Change activities or try to identify/anticipate the patient's needs in order to decrease frustration
- Patients with aphasia are at risk for Depression and Pseudobulbar Affect
- Consultation with a psychiatrist or Neuropsychiatrist for medication management may be necessary

Hegde, M. N. (1996). *PocketGuide to treatment in speech-language pathology*. San Diego, CA: Singular Publishing Group, Inc.

Apraxia. An inability to carry out purposeful or skilled movements to command by an individual who has normal motor functions (e.g., strength, tone, coordination, reflexes) and who has generally adequate auditory comprehension and intellectual skills.

- It is associated with left (dominant) hemisphere lesions and frequently accompanies Aphasia, which can make accurate assessment difficult when the patient's auditory comprehension is compromised
- The exact mechanisms of apraxia are not clearly understood although theories suggest that the left hemisphere is dominant for storing learned motor programs and for directing motor execution of the Right Hemisphere
- Visuokinetic motor engrams or programs (referred to as praxicons) are believed to be stored in the dominant parietal cortex and brain lesions may destroy the praxicons or result in a disconnection syndrome isolating the praxicons from the premotor or motor cortex in the Frontal Lobes

- There are several different types of apraxias (which are listed below) although the terminology can be confusing and is not used consistently throughout the field
- The examination of apraxia requires review of a variety of learned movements of the limbs, face, and body to imitation and to command (e.g., "Show me how you salute"), although there is no standard or widely accepted formal assessment procedure

Types of Apraxia

Ideomotor Apraxia. A disruption in the selection, sequencing, and spatial orientation of movements in response to a verbal command, especially involving a tool or object (e.g., "Show me how you would hammer a nail").

- Imitation from the examiner may improve the performance but it is frequently still defective
- Use of the actual object may also improve the performance of the patient, although not in all cases

Ideational Apraxia. This term has been used to describe an inability to carry out a sequence of acts in their proper order (e.g., wetting a facecloth, rinsing out the excess water, and putting on the soap) although each individual activity can be performed normally; this term has also been used to describe an inability to use the real or actual object, such as a comb, hammer, etc.

Buccofacial Apraxia. The inability to perform learned skilled movements of the face, lips, tongue, cheeks, larynx and pharynx on command; occurs in greater than 90% of patients with Broca's Aphasia; usually results from frontal or Corpus Callosum lesions.

Constructional Apraxia. Not likely a true apraxia, it refers to an inability to reproduce (copy) drawings or designs; it is frequently associated with deficits with Perceptual Functioning, including visual Neglect, Right Hemisphere syndromes, and in right Parietal Lobe damage; the patient's perceptual dysfunction, and not his or her motor programming, is likely most responsible for this impairment.

Dressing Apraxia. This, too, is not likely a true apraxia and is described as a problem dressing oneself due to an inability to orient clothing to one's own body; it is most common in Right Hemisphere syndromes and accompanies other deficits with Perceptual Functioning, however, left hemisphere lesions have also been known to cause this disorder, particularly if right/left disorientation is present; dressing apraxia is less common than constructional apraxia (approximately 1:4 ratio).

Treatment of Apraxia

- Hand-on-hand techniques may be necessary to assist the patient to complete motor acts
- Begin retraining proximal motor programs before distal movements are emphasized (e.g., use large arm movements before finger or fine motor functions)
- Encourage patients to approximate the correct movements even if they are not fully accurate
- Emphasize functional and overlearned tasks as part of therapy
- Teach compensatory strategies when appropriate
- Monitor frustration level as this may impede motivation in therapy and contribute to Depression

Heilman, K. M., & Gonzalez Rothi, L. J. (1993). Apraxia. In K. Heilman & E. Valenstein (Eds.), *Clinical neuropsychology* (3rd ed.), pp. 141–163. New York: Oxford University Press.

Mesulam, M. M. (1985). *Principles of behavioral neurology*. Philadelphia: F. A. Davis Co.

Aprosodia. A reduction or inability to use or appreciate the affective features of language; the patient cannot identify the emotional qualities of speech (i.e., anger, happiness, sarcasm, etc.); patients also cannot express emotions by the inflection and intonation in their speech; this can cause significant interpersonal problems and frustrations, given the importance of communicating emotions in *how* we speak; this disorder is the result of Right Hemisphere lesions.

Arachnoid Layer. A delicate avascular membrane below the Dura and above the Pia Mater; it is separated from the Dura by the Subdural space and from the Pia Mater by the Subarachnoid space.

Arithmetic Subtest. One of the subtests on the Wechlser Adult Intelligence Scale—Revised and the Wechsler Intelligence Scale for Children—III that assesses oral arithmetic and calculation skills.

Arousal. The state of wakefulness, Consciousness, or alertness of the individual, which can range from Coma to hypervigilance.

- Wakefulness is controlled neuroanatomically by the Reticular Activating System (RAS) in the Brain Stem and by the Thalamus
- Arousal level can be affected by many neuropathological conditions which affect the RAS, Thalamus, or both cerebral hemispheres; these may include Traumatic Brain Injury and subsequent Diffuse Axonal Injury, Cerebrovascular Accident, Tumor, metabolic encephalopathy, Anoxia, Hydrocephalus, and Seizures
- Changes in sleep, such as sleep apnea or nighttime insomnia, can affect arousal during the day (see Sleep Disorders)
- Adequate arousal is crucial for the patient to respond to the environment, maintain Attention, and participate in rehabilitation
- Descriptions of arousal levels differ among clinicians; listed here are some frequently used terms to describe arousal:
  - **Alert.** Awake and able to interact with the environment in a meaningful way
  - **Lethargic.** Not fully alert; tends to drift off to sleep; loses train of thought due to fatigue or decreased endurance; Attention and Memory are decreased

- **Stupor.** Responds only to persistent or vigorous stimulation; responses are minimal when awakened
- **Coma.** Unarousable (see Coma entry for more information)

Treatment of Arousal Problems in Rehabilitation

- Rule out ongoing medical condition, such as Hydrocephalus, or medication side effects/interactions that could account for impaired arousal and endurance
- Rule out Sleep Disorders or poor nighttime sleep; this may require careful monitoring of the patient's sleep pattern at night
- Assess for possible Depression
- Objectively record the patient's arousal level during the day (see following suggestions) by creating an "arousal monitor" to establish a baseline of the patient's ability to engage in therapy, to determine if any patterns emerge which may reflect when the patient is more or less awake, to assess which activities are most engaging for the patient, and to more objectively determine if arousal level is improving over time
  - Record the patient's arousal level for each 30-minute time period throughout the day by using a simple numerical rating system with which the treatment team feels comfortable; an example would be a 4-point rating scale with the following values: 4 = fully alert; 3 = easily arousable but tends to drift off to sleep; 2 = awake only with persistent stimulation; 1 = unarousable or barely arousable
  - For each 30-minute time period, the activity that the patient was involved with should also be recorded (e.g., table top activities in occupational therapy, in wheelchair in hall, in bed)
  - Whomever is with the patient during the 30-minute session should record the data; all treating staff need to be informed of this system and agree to participate
  - The "arousal monitor" must be kept with the patient at all times

  - The monitor should initially be put in place for a specified time period and then reviewed by the team at the end of that time; a decision to continue with the monitor would be made by the treatment team
  - Try to determine if a pattern exists; if the patient is more alert at certain times during the day or with certain activities, then plan treatment accordingly
- Provide rest breaks between therapies
- Schedule nap times during the day
- Consider co-treatments; two therapists working with the patient at one time may increase stimulation to keep the patient more alert
- When treating the patient be energetic, use increased volume and intonation/inflection in voice, and be enthusiastic about activities and exercises
- Try to engage the patient with topics of conversation, activities, music, or hobbies that are intrinsically meaningful to him or her; the family would need to be queried about this
- Increase the stimulation in the patient's environment for limited periods of time, such as seating him or her in the hall or near the nurse's station to assess the affect on arousal (note that interventions for arousal deficits, where efforts are designed to "draw out" or stimulate patients, are the opposite of treatment suggestions for <u>Agitation</u>, where the goal is to "contain" or minimize patient activity)
- Patient should engage in the most strenous activities (whether physical or cognitive) when most awake
- Encourage patient's family to observe and participate in treatment sessions; note the effect of their presence on the patient's arousal and alter their participation in treatment accordingly
- Save more enjoyable activities for the patient to participate in when the patient is slightly more fatigued or at the end of the session; the enjoyable task can be a reward or an incentive to persist when tired

- Establish an agreement with the patient (if cognitively able) that he or she can return to bed after completing specific therapeutic activities or after a previously agreed upon time period
- Frequently reorient the patient, explain why he or she is in the hospital, and the importance of participating in therapies
- When the patient is most awake and alert, assess the patient's cognitive status for basic functions such as Orientation, Attention, Awareness of injury, and Memory (address deficits in those areas as appropriate)
- As the patient's arousal improves, then Agitation may emerge as well as multiple cognitive deficits
- Consider use of psychostimulants if not medically contraindicated

Furie, K., & Feldmann, E. (1994). Disorders of consciousness. In E. Feldmann (Ed.), *Current diagnosis in neurology* (pp. 308–312). St. Louis, MO: Mosby-Year Book, Inc.

Strub, R. L., & Black, F. W. (1977). *The mental status examination in neurology*. Philadelphia, PA: F. A. Davis Co.

Arteriovenous Malformation (AVM). A congenital entanglement of blood vessels that forms an abnormal connection between veins and arteries; this results in an abnormal arterial-venous structure in place of a normal capillary bed.

- Most AVMs are asymptomatic and are relatively rare (approximately 2,000 new cases are identified each year in the U.S.)
- The most common first symptom of an AVM is a hemorrhage, usually an Intracerebral Hemorrhage rather than a Subarachnoid Hemorrhage because of the location of the AVM, although hemorrhages resulting from AVMs only comprise about 2–9% of all bleeds
- Hemorrhagic AVMs are most common during the second through fifth decades of life
- AVMs that do not present with hemorrhages, seizures, or other neurologic symptoms often do not produce focal

cognitive signs or deficits (likely due to the developmental nature of this anomaly which may result in cerebral organization that minimizes its effects); there may be some lateralizing signs, however, on neuropsychological testing

- Neurosurgical management of the AVM is required if symtomatic; the goal of treatment (surgery to remove or embolize the AVM or radiotherapy to eradicate or reduce it) is to stop blood flow through the AVM without damaging adjacent brain tissue or vessels
- The most significant cognitive deficits resulting from AVMs typically occur from the hemorrhages or surgical interventions

Brown, G. G., Spicer, K. B., & Malik, G. (1991). Neurobehavioral correlates of arteriovenous malformations and cerebral aneurysms. In R. A. Bornstein (Ed.), *Neurobehavioral aspects of cerebrovascular disease*. New York: Oxford University Press.

Astereognosis. The inability to identify an object by touch; sensitivity to the size, weight, and texture of the object may also be decreased; lesions generally in the area of the Parietal Lobes may result in this disorder.

Astrocytoma. A brain Tumor that arises from the astrocytes, one of two types of connective cells within the central nervous system (known as glial cells); astrocytomas are a common type of brain Tumor in children and tend to be located in the Cerebellum; in adults, astrocytomas are the most common primary brain tumor found; they are usually slow-growing initially but can grow more rapidly over time; most become symptomatic in the third or fourth decade (Seizures are the most common presenting symptom); they tend to infiltrate extensively into the gray and white matter of the Cerebrum and develop into more malignant forms, such as a Glioblastoma; with astrocytomas, a combination of surgery and radiotherapy may prolong life for 10 years.

Kaufman, D. M. (1995). *Clinical neurology for psychiatrists*. Philadelphia, PA: W. B. Saunders Co.

Brown, M. T., & Schold, S. C. (1994). Low-grade astrocytoma. In E. Feldmann (Ed.), *Current diagnosis in neurology* (pp. 134–137). St. Louis, MO: Mosby-Year Book, Inc.

Ataxia. An inability to coordinate muscles when executing voluntary movements; may affect limbs or gait; it results from damage to the Cerebellum or loss of proprioceptive sense in the extremities; can be associated with disorders such as Traumatic Brain Injury, Normal Pressure Hydrocephalus, Multiple Sclerosis, and Friedreich's Ataxia (a genetic disorder resulting in degeneration of the spinocerebellar tracts).

Atrophy, cerebral. A decrease in brain size or volume evident on CT and Magnetic Resonance Imaging (MRI) scans as widening sulci (the grooves on the brain's surface), narrowing gyri (the portions of brain lying between the sulci or grooves), thinning of the cortical mantle, and increasing ventricular size.

- It is a normal Aging Effect that may first become apparent in the 40s
- Atrophy is the result of neuronal loss, most notably in the Hippocampus, the Anterior portion of the Frontal Lobes, and in other selected Subcortical Structures, as well as a shrinkage in cell size
- Atrophy can be evident in older individuals who are functioning normally and in pathological conditions such as Dementia, in individuals with extensive Alcohol use, and as a sequelae to Traumatic Brain Injury
- In the elderly, atrophy alone is not diagnostic of a dementing disorder or of a deterioration in cognitive functions, as many older individuals with evidence of atrophy possess normal intellectual skills

Lezak, M. D. (1995). *Neuropsychological assessment* (3rd ed.). New York: Oxford University Press.

Attention. One of the most fundamental and basic (but complex) of all cognitive processes that refers generally to how individuals respond to or process stimuli in their environment.

- There is no unifying and definitive theory of attention and attentional disorders that is accepted by all clinicians and researchers although there is strong evidence that disorders of attention are common in a variety of insults to the central nervous system, particularly Traumatic Brain Injury and with Right Hemisphere and Frontal Lobe syndromes
- Attentional disorders can have a substantial impact on a patient's functioning across a wide range of activities and abilities, including activities of daily living, Memory (without proper attention, an individual will be unable to absorb or acquire new information), Problem Solving, social interactions, and vocational functioning
- Attention is highly dependent upon the patient's Arousal level, which is modulated by the Reticular Activating System and the Thalamus, although an individual can be fully alert and still exhibit a significant attentional disorder
- Frontal Lobe structures are also involved in the regulation and direction of attention
- Attention can also be affected by age, medications, endurance/fatigue, pain and physical discomfort, motivation, Delirium, and emotional or psychological factors such as Anxiety and Depression
- Mental Speed or rate of information processing is a related function to attention and is often impaired with attentional disorders
- The concept of Concentration is also related to attention but has no universally accepted definition; some may use the term interchangeably with focused or selective attention (see following definition); it may also be used to describe the ability to mentally manipulate information such as when performing mental calculations
- There are many constructs of attention but no universally accepted subtypes; research has suggested three basic components of attention:
  - The capacity to *focus* attention
  - The capacity to *sustain* attention
  - The capacity to *shift* attention

- The types of attention listed here are incorporated from the work of M. D. Lezak, and C. A. Mateer and R. L. Mapou; there may be significant overlap among the different subtypes of attention described

Subtypes of Attention

Immediate Attention Span. Refers to how much information the individual can grasp at any one moment or at one time; may also be referred to as working Memory (e.g., remembering a telephone number long enough to dial it).

Focused or Selective Attention. The ability to highlight or monitor the most important information or stimuli in the face of competing distractions (e.g., being able to listen to a conversation with the radio on or ambulate with a walker in a busy corridor without becoming distracted); incorporates the notion of distractibility.

Sustained Attention or Vigilance. To maintain attentional focus over an extended period of time (e.g., to be able to pay attention to a long set of instructions, a television show, to one's ADLs).

Divided Attention. The ability to respond to more than one task at a time or to multiple demands within the same activity (e.g., preparing a meal with more than one item or trying to perform ADLs at the sink while using a walker for support).

Alternating Attention. To be able to shift focus or attention between activities/tasks or ideas (e.g., the ability of patients to shift appropriately from one activity, such as brushing their teeth, to another activity, such as washing their face); the opposite of Perseveration.

Spatial Attention. The ability to visually scan the environment and to direct attention to the most salient stimuli in all visual fields; impairment in this domain is referred to as visual or spatial Neglect (see that entry for details on assessment and treatment) and is most associated with Right Hemisphere syndromes.

Assessment of Attention

- Observe the patient's behavior in a natural setting, as this is an important component in the assessment process
  - Does the patient orient or respond to you when you enter the room?
  - What is the patient's level of alertness or Arousal?
  - Is the patient able to focus on your questions and listen to explanations?
  - Is the patient distracted by external noises or other forms of stimulation?
  - How quickly does the patient respond to information or questions?
  - How well does the patient respond to multistep questions or instructions?
  - Is the patient able to shift his or her responses and behavior with the types of questions that are asked or with the demands of an activity?
  - Is the patient able to listen and respond to questions for an extended period of time or persist at a task until it is completed?
  - Does the presence of others, particularly family members, affect the patient's ability to initiate, attend, or persist at an activity?
  - If the patient has periods of inattention, ask him or her about what was happening during that period (i.e., did the patient forget what was happening or what he or she was asked to do, did the patient understand the instruction but didn't know how to do it, did the patient become distracted by his or her own thoughts or by things happening around him or her, etc.)
  - Is the patient aware of his or her attentional problems?
  - Does the patient become distracted by internal stimuli (his or her own thoughts) or by external stimuli (things in the environment)?
  - Other cognitive functions such as language, Memory, Problem Solving, and Executive Functions need to be

assessed; deficits in these areas can mimic or exacerbate attentional problems

- The use of objective and well-normed attentional measures is also a crucial part of the assessment process; listed here is a sample of some commonly used tests of attention:
  - The Wechsler Adult Intelligence Scale-Revised (WAIS-R) Digit Span, Arithmetic, and Digit Symbol subtests
  - The Attention/Concentration Index of the Wechsler Memory Scale—Revised
  - Many attentional tests are used routinely in neuropsychological batteries including Trail Making Test, Stroop Test, Symbol Digit Modalities Test, Seashore Rhythm Test, letter or symbol Cancellation Tests, and the Paced Auditory Serial Addition Test
  - Simple measures of mental control also assess attention and Concentration, some examples include performing mental calculations, reversing the days of the week, the months of the year, or the spelling of words
  - A Continuous Performance Test, of which there are many variations, is often used to assess sustained attention or vigilance
  - The Wisconsin Card Sorting Test is a multidimensional measure of cognitive functioning which also may assess the ability to remain on task or "in set" and to shift attention based upon environmental feedback
  - The Test of Everyday Attention is designed to assess attention under more natural conditions and activities
- Formal and objective assessment of attention as well as a determination of the patient's attention for more functional tasks are necessary for a comprehensive evalution of attention and for optimal treatment planning

Treatment of Attentional Disorders

- Rule out or treat other cognitive deficits, particularly Aphasia, Memory disorders, and Executive Function deficits
- Rule out or treat psychological conditions that may be interfering with attention such as Depression or Anxiety

- Assist patients in developing better Awareness of their attentional problems so that they may anticipate when and under which circumstances their inattention may interfere with their functional abilities (if patients can anticipate problems then they are more likely to use strategies to compensate for them)
- Treatment suggestions will be grouped by whether they are clinician, environmental, or patient-centered (specific Cognitive Rehabilition exercises are listed at the end of this section)
- The following interventions for attentional problems are *clinician-centered* (i.e., techniques that the clinician can do or behavior that the clinician can exhibit to help patients with their attentional functions):
  - Keep instructions brief and in simple language
  - Make sure the patient has established eye contact with you before speaking
  - Use the patient's name frequently
  - Try to maintain eye contact with the patient while talking with him or her and encourage the patient to do the same (avoid eye contact, however, if the patient finds this too distracting)
  - Try to stand or sit in front of the patient at his or her eye level
  - Give only one instruction or bit of information at a time
  - Slow down rate of speech
  - Redirect the patient back to the task as necessary with verbal prompts or gestures
  - Present information in an organized and hierarchical fashion from the simple to the more complex
  - Repeat information as necessary
  - Use the appropriate tone of voice (if patients are distractible then a loud voice may interfere with their ability to attend but if they are underaroused then more intonation and louder volume may be helpful)
  - Limit choices for the patient—be more directive

- Explain the purpose of the task that you are asking patients to perform and how it relates to their rehabilitation needs
- Touch the patient lightly, if necessary, to direct his or her attention to the task or instructions being given
- Prompt or cue the patient to attend by statements such as "I have something important to say . . ." or "I want you to really pay attention to this . . ."
- Give patient time to process information before giving the next instruction or moving on to the next activity
- Shorten treatment sessions if fatigue interferes with attentional functions
- Give the most cognitively demanding tasks earlier in the day when endurance problems and fatigue are less prominent
- Break tasks into smaller units
- Give only one activity to perform at a time
- Provide patients with concrete feedback, both positive and negative, about their performance
- Socially praise patients for those periods when they are being attentive, if only for a few minutes (be specific about how you observed their improved attention and why it is important that they continue to work on this problem)
- Acknowledge patients' attempts at taking a more active role in monitoring and improving their attention (e.g., reinforce the patient who comments, "Can you close that door because the noise in the hall is bothering me")
- Describe to patients what you observe about their "inattentive behaviors" (e.g., looking around the room, playing with an article of their clothing, talking while transfering)
- Meet as a team to discuss what techniques are most effective in treating the patient

• The following interventions are *environmentally centered* techniques (i.e., changes that are made to the environment to help patients with their attentional deficits):

- Treat in a distraction-free environment
- Keep extraneous stimulation, both auditory and visual, to a minimum (avoid "clutter" in the room)
- Try to have the same clinicians treating the patient on a daily basis
- When performing ADLs, give the patient only one article of clothing or one item (e.g., toothbrush, shaver) at a time
- Keep and store objects of similar use together (e.g., group together objects used for grooming and keep them separate from other, nonrelated objects)
- Monitor environmental stimuli such as temperature, lighting, etc., as they may increase or decrease attentional functions
- Consider co-treatments if it does not increase the patient's distractibility (sometimes with co-treatments one therapist can be working on a specific movement while the other therapist is monitoring and encouraging attentional functions)
- Determine if your presence in the patient's line of sight is distracting
- Use brightly colored stimuli to engage the patient's attention
- Try to engage the patient in his or her premorbid interests and hobbies
- Limit the number of visitors if their presence is too distracting
- Use incentives to improve attention (e.g., if the patient can complete a task accurately within a specific time period then he or she can go to bed for a rest)
- Gradually increase the task demands and the amount of distracting stimuli in the environment as the patient can tolerate it
- Educate and involve the family in how to interact with the patient
- Consider the use of psychostimulants to increase attentional functions

- The following interventions are *patient-centered* techniques (e.g., the clinician is asking something of the patient and is making him or her a more active agent in the treatment process)
  - Ask patients what thoughts, if any, are interfering with their ability to pay attention (e.g., family visiting, discharge date, fear of falling) and then try to address these issues as best as possible
  - Ask patients to predict how attentive they think they will be during an activity and then after the activity ask them how they think they did (to be used to assess and improve patient's insight and Awareness of their attentional abilities)
  - Ask the patient to check his or her own work after completion
  - Have patients repeat instructions to ensure that they were attending when they were first given
  - If a patient suddenly becomes inattentive, ask the patient if he or she was aware of the attentional lapse and what he or she was thinking of at that time
  - Begin with a specific baseline about how well the patient can attend to a particular stimulus and then encourage and challenge him or her to improve his or her performance if only by a small percentage every day (e.g., "You were able to keep your eyes focused on this ball for 12 seconds yesterday, let's see if you can increase that to 15 seconds today")
  - Keep a record of the patient's performance on attentional tasks, post it in the patient's room, refer to it at every therapy session, and use it as an incentive (and reward) to improve
  - Set a time limit on how long it should take a patient to complete a specific task accurately
  - Videotape a patient performing a task and review with him or her
  - Have the patient verbally prompt him- or herself to attend by saying aloud "focus" or "pay attention" prior

to beginning an activity (the verbal prompt can be gradually faded to the patient saying it silently to him- or herself)

- Encourage good posture to improve alertness

- The following Cognitive Rehabilitation techniques may also be effective in the remediation of attention problems (begin with exercises that the patient is able to accomplish and gradually increase the difficulty as the patient is able to tolerate it):
  - *Time estimation exercises*: Ask patients to estimate how long 10, 15, and 60 second time intervals have passed; suggest techniques to help them monitor the passage of time intervals by tapping their feet, nodding their heads, etc.; use this type of activity to demonstrate the efficiency or inefficiency of their attention as attentional problems will create significant over- or underestimates of the passage of time
  - *Visual vigilance tasks*: These activities require patients to sustain their attention over an extended time to repetitive visual stimuli; an example of this exercise would be to slowly show playing cards to the patient one at a time and ask the patient to knock on the table each time a red card is shown—the demands can be easily increased, both with regard to rate of presentation and complexity (the patient could be asked to respond each time a red face card is shown, if a red card is immediately preceded by a black card, etc.)
  - *Auditory vigilance tasks*: These activities require the patient to attend to stimuli that are presented auditorially; for example, patients could be asked to signal the examiner each time a target letter, number, or word is said from a list of alternatives; the complexity can be magnified by increasing the rate of presentation (e.g., reading the stimuli at faster speeds) or by changing the stimuli the patient is asked to respond to (e.g., signaling only to words beginning with vowels)

- *Reaction time exercises*: In this exercise the patient must respond to a single stimulus as quickly as possible (computer-based exercises can be helpful in this area because the presentation of and the time to respond to the stimulus can be controlled and measured precisely)
- *Visual tracking tasks*: These tasks require the patient to cross out or find stimuli presented on a page, such as visually searching for a specific letter or symbol in rows of random letters or symbols (see Cancellation Tasks)
- *Mental control activities*: In these activities the patient must perform mental operations such as calculations, reversing sequences of numbers or letters, etc.
- *Mental shifting tasks*: An example of this activity would be to show the patient a list of numbers, have him or her write the number that would come after the number on the paper, then for the next number write the number that would come before it

- Attention retraining programs (some computer assisted) are available; see below for selected references

Ben-Yishay, Y., Piasetsky, E. B., & Rattock, J. (1987). A systematic method for ameliorating disorders in basic attention. In M. Meyer, A. Benton, and L. Diller (Eds.), *Neuropsychological rehabilitation*. Edinburgh: Churchill Livingstone.

Gansler, D. A., & McCaffrey, R. J. (1991). Remediation of chronic attention deficits in traumatic brain-injured patients. *Archives of Clinical Neuropsychology, 6*, 335–353.

Lezak, M. D. (1995). *Neuropsychological assessment* (3rd ed.). New York: Oxford University Press.

Mateer, C. A., & Mapou, R. L. (1996). Understanding, evaluating, and managing attention disorders following brain injury. *Journal of Head Trauma Rehabilitation, 11*, 1–16.

Mirsky, A. F., Anthony, B. J., Duncan, C. C., Ahearn, M. B., & Kellam, S. G. (1991). Analysis of the elements of attention: A neuropsychological approach. *Neuropsychology Review, 2*, 109–145.

Sohlberg, M. M., Johnson, L., Paule, L., Raskin, S. A., & Mateer, C. M. (1993). *Attention process training—II: A program to address attentional deficits for persons with mild cognitive dysfunction.* Puyallup, WA: Association for Neuropsychological Research and Development.

Sohlberg, M. M., & Mateer, C. A. (1986). *Attention process training (APT)*. Puyallup, WA: Association for Neuropsychological Research and Development.

Whyte, J. (1992). Neurologic disorders of attention and arousal: Assessment and treatment. *Archives of Physical Medicine and Rehabilitation, 73*, 1094–1103.

Attention Deficit Hyperactivity Disorder (ADHD). A persistent pattern of inattention and/or hyperactivity-impulsivity that is more frequent or severe than typically seen in individuals of comparable ages.

- The symptoms must have been present since childhood, with some symptoms evident before the age of 7
- The symptoms must interfere with the person's functioning in at least two settings (i.e., home, school, or community)
- Some of the symptoms of ADHD decrease with age, particularly the excessive hyperactivity, and may remit completely by or after adolescence, although some persons' symptoms may persist in some form in adulthood
- The current term of ADHD replaces what was formerly known as Attention Deficit Disorder (ADD) with or without hyperactivity
- An individual may now be diagnosed with one of three variations of the disorder—ADHD Predominantly Inattentive Type (i.e., inattentive but not hyperactive), ADHD Predominantly Hyperactive-Impulsive type (i.e., hyperactive but not inattentive), and ADHD Combined Type (i.e., inattentive and hyperactive)
- Children with ADHD may be at higher risk for sustaining brain injuries than children without ADHD due to impulsive behavior and risk-taking
- There is a higher rate of school failure, behavioral problems, substance abuse, antisocial behaviors, and Learning Disabilities with children with ADHD than without
- ADHD is usually treated with a combination of environmental/behavioral interventions and psychostimulant medication such as Ritalin

- It is important to query patients with TBI and their family members for evidence of ADHD as this will provide important information about the patient's baseline level of functioning and will provide some expectations for postinjury behavior that may be unrelated to the injury
- Problems with Attention are very common following brain injury although when they are the result of trauma later in life they should not be referred to as ADHD
- The behavioral characteristics listed here are a sample of symptoms of inattention and impulsivity-hyperactivity from the ADHD diagnostic criteria in the *Diagnostic and Statistical Manual of Mental Disorders* (4th edition):
  - *Inattention*: makes careless mistakes; doesn't seem to listen when spoken to; has problems organizing activities; loses things; easily distracted
  - *Impulsivity-hyperactivity*: fidgets or squirms; talks too much; interrupts others; has problems awaiting turn; acts as if "driven by a motor"

Autobiographical Memory. A measure of long-term or remote Memory of the individual's personal history.

- Some data may be easy to verify such as home address, date of birth, and names and ages of immediate family members, although other information may be more difficult to confirm such as the year the patient got married, educational or occupational history, etc.
- This type of Memory is the most resistant to deterioration following brain trauma
- Amnesia for autobiographical information may occur during acute recovery from some disorders such as Traumatic Brain Injury, Anoxia, Herpes Simplex Encephalitis, or Subarachnoid Hemorrhages although the Amnesia is usually for events that happened in the more recent past rather than for events that happened longer ago (e.g., patients may be unable to remember their home address of the last 10 years but may recall their home address from childhood, or they may believe that their adult chil-

dren are much younger than they actually are)—this Amnesia usually improves

- In nearly all cases, autobiographical Memory deficits are accompanied by severe short-term Memory deficits or Anterograde Amnesia
- Some disorders, such as Korsakoff's Syndrome and Alzheimer's Disease, may result in a permanent deficit for autobiographical Memory, and with Alzheimer's Disease this impairment will worsen with time

Automatisms. Simple, repetitive, and purposeless movements such as lip-smacking, kissing, scratching/rubbing clothes or the body; associated with partial complex Seizures.

Awareness. The ability to appreciate one's impairments; the level of insight that patients have in understanding the nature of their deficits, including the need for treatment and their affects on daily functioning.

- Awareness is a crucial variable in a patient's rehabilitation that must be assessed and treated as part of the Cognitive Rehabilitation program
- Awareness facilitates a patient's participation in rehabilitation, the willingness to use compensatory strategies, to accept performance feedback, to make safe judgments, and to interact appropriately with others
- A lack of awareness can be the result of psychological denial, which is an emotional reaction to the injury or disability, a neurologically (organic) based unawareness, known as Anosognosia, or a combination of both
  - Psychological denial tends to emerge later in the recovery process, may be related to premorbid Personality factors and coping methods, and is not related to any specific syndrome of neurologic impairments or to lesions in any particular brain area
  - Anosognosia usually occurs during the acute recovery period (although it may persist to some degree indefinitely), is often associated with confusion and problems with Orientation, may occur more frequently with

greater cognitive deficits, and is generally most common in Right Hemisphere lesions, Dementia, and Traumatic Brain Injury

- Unawareness may be limited to specific areas of functioning but not to others; for example, patients may be unaware of cognitive disturbances but aware of hemiplegia (the converse is almost never true) or aware of cognitive problems but unaware of Personality changes
- Patients may acknowledge some of their deficits, such as weakness or Memory problems, but may be unaware of their impact on their safety, ability to function on a day-to-day basis, the need to use compensatory aids, or their ability to return to work
- Unawareness of cognitive deficits may be evident in up to 90% of acute Right Hemisphere CVAs (Anderson & Tranel, 1989)
- One study (Oddy, Coughlan, Tyerman, & Jenkins, 1985) revealed that seven years after, TBI family members reported that 40% of patients "refused to admit difficulties"; unawareness in TBI may be related to bilateral lesions or Frontal Lobe damage, particularly for social awareness
- The relationship between self-report of cognitive functioning and actual abilities is generally weak
- An Awareness Interview has been reported to help quantify the discrepancy between a patient's report of abilities and objective assessment of those abilities

Treatment of Awareness Deficits

- There is no single, well-validated method of remediating awareness deficits; treatment consists of a multifaceted, consistent team approach to improving insight
- Decide which exact words will be used to tell patients what happened to them (for example, if a patient has suffered a head injury and Subdural Hematoma in a motor vehicle accident the patient may be told by one person that he or she was in a car accident, may be told by anoth-

er that there was bleeding in the brain, or by someone else that he or she had a head injury—all these different explanations to a confused person will not increase awareness as to why he or she is in the hospital); the treatment team must therefore decide which specific reason will be given (and which exact words will be used) to explain the necessity for hospitalization; this precise explanation must be used by all treating clinicians and the patient's family

- The patient's injury, deficits, their functional implications, and treatment are all interconnected and need to be reviewed with the patient repeatedly in order to increase knowledge of his or her condition
  - Write down for the patient the two to four most serious cognitive impairments resulting from the injury that interfere most with daily functioning; use brief explanations that the patient can understand (e.g., "You have problems remembering things") and review this list with the patient several times during treatment
  - Describe to the patient in simple language how these problems or deficits interfere with daily functioning (e.g., "Because of your problems remembering things you forget to take your medication")
  - Explain to the patient that treatment is related to his or her deficits (e.g., "Because of your problems with your Memory and taking your pills you will need to learn how to use a Memory book")
  - Reinforce and review with patients the interconnection among their deficits, the functional implications of their deficits, the need for treatment, and that all these factors are the result of their injury or the reason for their hospitalization (use whatever words were agreed on by the team to explain to the patient what happened to him or her)
  - The goal is for patients to be able to appreciate the cause and nature of their problems, the need for treat-

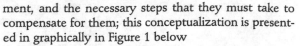

ment, and the necessary steps that they must take to compensate for them; this conceptualization is presented in graphically in Figure 1 below

- Give patients concrete and very specific feedback about their performance and how their deficits are related to their injury or reason for hospitalization; refer them back to their problem list (described previously) that was written down for them; use examples such as, "When you turned to see who was walking by you almost lost your balance. That is an example of your problem with paying attention that we wrote down for you; the problem is caused by the injury to your brain"; the exact type and specificity of the feedback will need to be modified depending upon the patient's cognitive functioning
- Although methods at improving insight tend to highlight only the patients' problems, the manner in which these

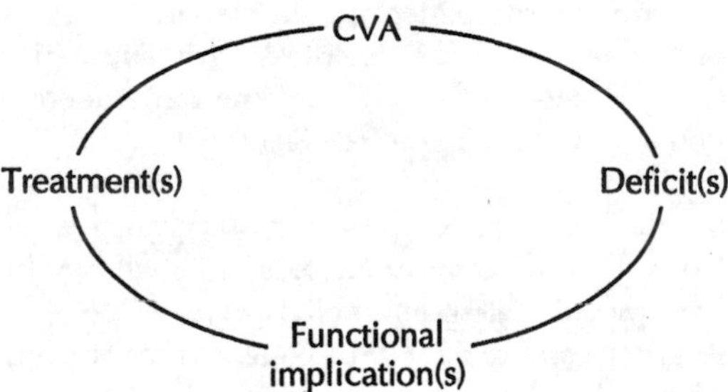

Figure 1. Model of communication to increase patient insight. (Reprinted with permission from Neurocognitive Rehabilitation Guidelines for Therapists by T. J. Guilmette and M. L. Kennedy, 1995, p. 35. *Topics in Stroke Rehabilitation: Family and Other Psychological Issues,* 2(2). Copyright 1995 Aspen Publishers, Inc.)

problems or deficits are communicated to patients need to consider their emotional state (i.e., patients can be partially unaware of their deficits and depressed simultaneously, which would modulate how forcefully their impairments would be communicated to them in order to not increase their dysphoria and poor self-esteem)

- Use words, language, vocabulary, and examples that patients can understand and that are consistent with their education and cultural backgrounds
- For patients who are completely unaware of their condition, a first step is to help them at least repeat or parrot back what is wrong with them (even if they don't believe it)
- Establish a trusting relationship with the patient as this may help the patient more easily accept the feedback he or she is receiving (i.e., why should patients who are convinced that they have no problems believe someone that they don't know tell them otherwise?)
- Educate family members and close friends about the nature and cause of the patient's insight problems; encourage them to explain and reinforce to the patient his or her problems and need for treatment using the same language agreed upon by the team
- Conduct cognitive and neuropsychological assessments to determine the patient's relative strengths and weaknesses
- Explain to patients that their injury itself makes it hard for them to recognize their own problems (i.e., that the part of the brain that was injured "plays tricks" on them by not letting them see themselves accurately)
- Ask patients to predict their performance before they attempt an activity and then ask them to review it again after it has been completed; review how close they came to their prediction and to their appraisal of their own functioning
- Gently confront patients with the discrepancy between their beliefs about their functioning and how they are actually performing in treatment

- Continue to give hope to patients by asserting that in spite of their problems their functioning can improve with treatment
- Keep a log book of progress and problem areas, especially for those patients with Memory deficits
- Review with patients the specific abilities or skills that they will need to demonstrate before progressing to a higher level of functioning (e.g., to be discharged home, independent in their room, return to work)
  - Attempt to have patients agree to this list of concrete and observable skills that they will need to demonstrate in order to progress to their desired goal (e.g., take all medication correctly for 3 days in a row without cueing, walk 25 feet three times between 8: 00 AM and 3: 00 PM without any physical assistance needed)
  - Write down these concrete and observable skills in a checklist format and post in the patient's room
  - When the skill or ability on the list is demonstrated by the patient it can be be checked off
  - Encourage the patient's family to support this procedure
  - If patients are unable to perform the activities previously agreed on, do not argue with patients over their rationalizations about why they couldn't complete the activities (patients may rationalize that they didn't have the time to do the activities, they could have done them if they were home, they didn't feel well, etc.), simply keep them focused on the list of the skills they must demonstrate and how therapy will assist them in improving those abilities
- Videotape the patient performing an activity that demonstrates his or her problems and then review with the patient; this needs to be done cautiously as this direct confrontation may increase resistance or Depression
- For problems with social awareness and Personality changes, group therapy may be of benefit (see Social Skills Training)

Anderson, S. W., & Tranel, D. (1989). Awareness of disease states following cerebral infarction, dementia, and head trauma: Standardized assessment. *The Clinical Neuropsychologist, 3*, 327–339.

Guilmette, T. J., & Kennedy, M. L. (1995). Neurocognitive rehabilitation guidelines for therapists. *Topics in Stroke Rehabilitation, 2*, 32–43.

Oddy, M., Coughlan, T., Tyerman, A., & Jenkins, D. (1985). Social adjustment after closed head injury: A further follow-up seven years after injury. *Journal of Neurology, Neurosurgery, and Psychiatry, 48*, 564–568.

Prigatano, G. P., & Altman, I. M. (1990). Impaired awareness of behavioral limitations after traumatic brain injury. *Archives of Physical Medicine and Rehabilitation, 71*, 1058–1064.

Awareness Interview. A standardized interview that elicits from patients descriptions of their condition and Awareness of their reason for hospitalization, motor impairments, Orientation problems, cognitive impairments, Memory and speech problems, perceptual difficulties, and their ability to return to normal activities; patients' responses are compared with their actual abilities in each of the domains.

Anderson, S. W., & Tranel, D. (1989). Awareness of disease states following cerebral infarction, dementia, and head trauma: Standardized assessment. *The Clinical Neuropsychologist, 3*, 327–339.

Axon. The part of the neuron (nerve cell) that sends information from the cell body to other neurons (see Diffuse Axonal Injury); also referred to as White Matter due to the white covering of the axon by the myelin sheath which increases the efficiency of nerve conduction.

Babinski Response. When the lateral aspect of the sole of the foot is stroked, the normal response is flexion of the toes, but when the Babinski Response (which is abnormal after the age of 2) is present, the great toe will dorsiflex and the other toes will fan; this indicates an upper motor neuron lesion (i.e., above the level of the spinal cord).

Balint's Syndrome. A visuoperceptual disorder that impairs the ability of a person to perceive the visual field as a whole; it is composed of three components and is usually related to bilateral damage of the occipitoparietal region:

- *Simultanagnosia:* the inability to grasp the entire field of vision; the person can see clearly only a fraction of what is in front of him or her and that fragment may move or shift from view
- *Optic Ataxia:* the inability to accurately point to a target using visual guidance only
- *Ocular Apraxia:* the inability to direct one's gaze toward an object in the peripheral visual field

Ballismus. Intermittent flinging or violent movements of the arm and/or leg on one side of the body; usually associated with damage to the contralateral subthalamic nucleus.

Basal Ganglia. A group of structures located at the base of the cerebral hemispheres composed of the corpus striatum (Caudate Nucleus and the putamen), the globus pallidus, and the substantia nigra; these structures are interconnected and project pathways to and from the Frontal Lobes; lesions to the Basal Ganglia commonly result in movement disorders such as Parkinson's Disease and Huntington's Disease given the role of the Basal Ganglia in modulating and sequencing complex voluntary movements; the Basal Ganglia may also play a role in Procedural Learning and lesions have been reported to disrupt language functions (left side), spatial Attention (right side), and Personality functioning including Agitation and Abulia (bilateral damage); see Subcortical Structures.

Basilar Artery. The artery formed by the joining of the two Vertebral Arteries at the base of the brain (Brain Stem); it supplies blood to the Brain Stem, Cerebellum, and to the Posterior portions of the cerebral hemispheres; strokes in the basilar artery can result in Cranial Nerve abnormalities, Transient Global Amesia, Ataxia, and Vertigo; see Circle of Willis and Cerebral Circulation.

Beck Depression Inventory. A 21-item, self-report measure of depressive symptomatology widely used in clinical practice, particularly with outpatients; the scale contains 7 items that tap physical or somatic complaints (e.g., weight loss, sleep problems) which may limit its use with neurologic and elderly populations.

Beck, A. T. (1987). *Beck Depression Inventory.* San Antonio, TX: The Psychological Corporation.

Behavior Contracts. An agreement or "contract" usually established between the patient and the treatment team that specifies in observable and measurable terms what behaviors the patient will exhibit (usually what specific tasks the patient will perform in treatment) and what the consequences of fulfilling the contract will be, such as remaining in treatment, using the telephone, etc.

- Contracts may be most helpful for patients whose emotional or Personality functioning interfere with treatment (e.g., individuals who are controlling and do not accept direction well, passive-aggressive personalities, and those who are ambivalent about treatment which results in questionable compliance and Motivation)
- Contracting is meant to improve patient compliance and may help reduce the emotional friction or tension between patients and treating therapists, the latter of whom may feel that each treatment session is a struggle to motivate the patient to perform activities that he or she is capable of exhibiting

- Assess and treat emotional problems that may interfere with the patient's focus in rehabilitation such as Depression or Anxiety
- The patient must actively participate in drawing up the contract with a member of the treatment team who has the best relationship with the patient; do not be judgmental or moralizing when establishing the parameters of the contract, it should be presented in a "matter of fact" manner; explain that the agreement will help everyone understand the expectations for treatment
- The behaviors that the patient agrees to perform must be observable, measurable, and unambiguous (e.g., perform 25 straight leg raises twice per day during physical therapy)
- The contract may also include limits on what the therapists can ask the patient to do (e.g., walk no more than a specific distance, stay out of bed for no more than a specified period of time); this may help the patient feel that the treatment team is also making accommodations and compromises
- The contract should be for a limited period of time and should be renegotiated at the end of the time period (the new behaviors that the patient is expected to exhibit should be increased to reflect the patient's improvement since the previous agreement)
- The support of the patient's family is very important for the success of this type of intervention
- Patients must be at a high enough level cognitively to appreciate the demands of the agreement and the consequences for not complying
- The contract should be written out and signed by the patient and a member of the treatment team
- Post the contract in the patient's room so that the patient and the treating therapists can refer to it frequently
- If necessary a daily checklist can be made part of the contract so that each behavior that the patient has agreed to exhibit can be recorded daily

- Once the contract is in place do not "argue" with patients about why they may have not complied (if they have not) or "cajole" patients into participating with treatment; the contract alone should serve as the standard for patient participation; in a nonjudgmental fashion continually refer patients back to their agreement and its consequences

Behavior Management. The use of behavioral principles and interventions (e.g., reward, reinforcement, Extinction) designed to increase appropriate behaviors and decrease unwanted or inappropriate behaviors.

- Behavior management techniques are most often used in the treatment of socially inappropriate behaviors such as Agitation and Disinhibition as well as general impairments of daily functioning such as Abulia
- Although the primary cause of behavior disorders following brain injury is believed to be organic or biologically based, environmental factors such as Antecedents to the behavior (e.g., frustation, criticism) and consequences of the behavior (e.g., increased attention, getting one's way, avoiding unpleasant circumstances) can increase the likelihood of initiating and maintaining the presence of inappropriate behaviors
- The patient's premorbid Personality and emotional functioning will also have some effect on the postinjury behavior of the individual
- A combination of behavior management techniques and pharmacologic intervention may be necessary for severe behavioral problems
- See related entries such as Agitation, Behavior Contracts, Social Skills Training, and Awareness

Principles of Behavior Management

- Behavior management plans need to be highly individualized to the patient—there is no "cookbook" approach for every problem or patient

- Behavioral interventions are labor intensive and require very consistent interventions and approaches to patient care (they require time to set up, monitor, and readjust)
- All treating therapists, staff, and family must be in agreement about the goals of the program and the interventions that are prescribed
- Neuropsychological assessment is recommended to better understand the patient's cognitive strengths and weaknesses, which will provide guidance about how to instruct and teach the patient alternate behaviors
- Rewarding or reinforcing appropriate behaviors is generally more effective than punishing or extinguishing inappropriate behaviors
- Define in concrete, observable, and quantifiable terms the behavior being targeted for change
  - It must be measurable and specific (e.g., "Aggression" is not measurable but hitting, swearing, and kicking are)
  - If the patient does not have Awareness of his or her own behavior problem, then treatment must also include increasing insight (see Awareness entry for details)
  - The patient's family needs to be supportive and included in the program
- Analyze the Antecedents of the behavior (i.e., what happens in the patient's environment or what do other people do that increase or decrease the target behavior?)
  - Anticipate the Antecedents of the unwanted behavior and change environmental conditions if possible
  - Help patients recognize and anticipate the Antecedents to their inappropriate behavior; teach them methods to respond more appropriately or avoid situations that result in loss of control
  - Educate family members about behavioral Antecedents and what they can do to modify them (e.g., if their tone of voice increases the patient's Agitation, then they also need to learn to change how they talk with the patient)

- Analyze the consequences of the target behavior (i.e., what happens to the patient or in his or her environment after the target behavior is exhibited?)
- Establish a baseline of how frequently the target behavior occurs (this may be established for any time interval—minutes, hours, days, etc.) or fails to occur (such as not performing ADLs)
- Develop a plan to reward appropriate behaviors, such as initiating ADLs, taking medications, speaking in a normal tone of voice, etc., and/or extinguish inappropriate ones, such as swearing, hitting others, etc.
- Examples of rewards/reinforcements for appropriate behaviors:
  - Base rewards on the patient's history, interests, etc., not on what the team thinks should be reinforcing
  - A reward or reinforcer is by definition any response to a behavior that increases the likelihood that the behavior will be exhibited again or repeated (if the reward system is not increasing the frequency of the target behavior, then the reward is not powerful enough and the team must establish a new reinforcer)
  - Social reinforcement such verbal praise, spending time with the patient, smiling, a pat on the back, etc. can be powerful
  - Tangible reinforcers such as videos, television time, snacks, etc. may be appropriate
  - A <u>Token Economy</u> in which appropriate behaviors are rewarded with tokens that the patient can later "trade in" for other tangible rewards (most difficult system to use due to the high degree of coordination and planning required)
- Make liberal use of verbal praise in reinforcing patients' positive behaviors, no matter how small
  - Praise frequently patients' positive behaviors and give them concrete feedback about what they are doing prop-

erly and why it is important (we tend to only respond to negative behaviors)

- Use their names when giving feedback
- Make eye contact when talking with patients
- Smile when giving feedback
- Give patients a reassuring touch on the arm, a pat on the back, etc.
- Speak in a positive tone of voice and use words patients can understand
- Do not talk down or in a patronizing way to patients
- The praise should come immediately after the behavior is exhibited

- Methods of extinguishing inappropriate behaviors:
    - Tell patient to "stop" and label in concrete terms the behavior that is inappropriate (do not be judgmental and do not lecture)
    - Withdraw social contact, turn away, or ignore patient
    - The withdrawal of social contact must be immediate
    - Long "time out" periods are not necessary; 30 seconds to a few minutes can be sufficient
- Ignore inappropriate behaviors if they do not harm or threaten persons or property (this too is a method of Extinction); when undesirable behaviors are ignored they often initially increase in frequency but later subside
- Other negative consequences to behavioral problems can be used such as taking away privileges like the telephone, snacks, etc.; this is a form of punishment that should be used very judiciously as it tends to be less effective than rewarding appropriate behavior
- When "correcting" patients' behaviors, give them examples of more appropriate responses and ask them to practice (then verbally praise or reinforce the correct behavior)
- Be empathetic and acknowledge that it is difficult for the patient to control his or her behavior
- Pay close attention to how the patient is responding emotionally to the behavioral program; be careful not to empha-

size only the negative things the patient is or is not doing; balance feedback with concrete examples of the things the patient does well

- Acknowledge the patient's effort, persistence, and desire, not just the result
- Teach effective alternatives to patients' inappropriate behavior, have them practice more appropriate behaviors, give them feedback about their performance, and review why changing their behavior is important
- Reward improvement and remind patients of gains
- Do not show anger or disrespect to patients
- Avoid global, nonspecific comments about behavior such as "stop doing it like that" or "do it right" (these comments do not teach the patient anything)
- Evaluate results; compare the efficacy of the program with the baseline established prior to the onset of the intervention

Blackerby, W. F., & Gualtieri, T. (1991). Recent advances in neurobehavioral rehabilitation. *NeuroRehabilitation, 1*, 53–61.

Burke, W. H., & Wesolowski, H. D. (1988). Applied behavioral analysis in head injury rehabilitation. *Rehabilitation Nursing, 13*, 186–188.

Benton Visual Retention Test (BVRT). A measure of visual Memory or a Memory-for-designs test with three alternative forms and four different methods of administration; it is used with both children and adults; it is sensitive to Dementia and to other types of neurologic disorders that result in Memory impairments.

Sivan, A. B. (1995). *Benton Visual Retention Test Manual* (5th ed.). New York, NY: The Psychological Corporation.

Block Design. One of the 11 subtests from the Wechsler Adult Intelligence Scale—Revised and the Wechsler Intelligence Scale for Children—III; it is a measure of Constructional Ability that requires the person to replicate with red and white blocks patterns from a model or a picture; it is generally most sensitive to right Posterior lesions, particularly in the Parietal Lobe; Block Design is also vulnerable to the effects of Aging, chronic Alcohol use, and Dementia.

Boston Diagnostic Aphasia Exam (BDAE). A test battery used for the assessment of language functions and Aphasia in adults; it is composed of 34 subtests assessing 12 general areas of communication.

Boston Naming Test (BNT). Used to assess confrontation naming in which the patient is shown 60 ink drawings and is asked to name the pictures; a measure of Anomia.

Bradykinesia. Slowed physical movements.

Bradyphrenia. Slowed Mental Speed or rate of information processing; the cognitive equivalent to Bradykinesia; usually associated with illnesses such as Parkinson's Disease involving Subcortical brain structures but can be evident in many neuropathological conditions including Traumatic Brain Injury, Dementia, and medication side effects; see Attention.

Brain Stem. The lowest and farthest back portion of the brain; it is composed of three basic divisions (from lowest to highest): Medulla, Pons, and Midbrain; it connects the cerebral hemispheres with the spinal cord and contains basic life-sustaining centers for respiration, blood pressure, and heart rate; the Cranial Nerves and the Reticular Activating System are contained in the Brain Stem; lesions can produce Coma, Cranial Nerve damage such as Diplopia, and Nystagmus; unless Arousal levels are affected, damage to the Brain Stem usually leaves higher cognitive functions intact.

Bulbar Nerves. A group of Cranial Nerves (IX through XII) which originate from the area of the bulb (Medulla) in the Brain Stem and innervate muscles necessary for talking and swallowing (i.e., the muscles of the soft palate, pharynx, larynx, and tongue); lesions to these nerves can result in a bulbar palsy characterized by Dysarthria and Dysphagia.

California Verbal Learning Test (CVLT). An objective measure of verbal learning and Memory in which the person is read a list of 16 shopping items (composed of four items in each of four categories) over five learning trials; the person then is read an interfering list of 16 different items and is asked to recall the original list; after a 30-minute delay the person is asked to first spontaneously recall the original 16 items and then to recognize them from a longer list; this test is sensitive to verbal Memory deficits from such neurologic disorders as Dementia and Traumatic Brain Injury.

Delis, D. C., Kramer, J., Kaplan, E., Ober, B. A., & Fridlund, A. (1987). *The California Verbal Learning Tes*t New York: Psychological Corporation.

Cancellation Tests. Tests in which the patient is asked to scan a paper and cross out (or cancel) specific target stimuli; the stimuli may be letters, symbols, or shapes and may be arranged in rows or randomly placed on the page; there are other distracting stimuli interspersed with the targets; used to assess visual scanning, organization, planning, and Neglect.

Capgras Syndrome. A fixed Delusion or belief that a person or persons (usually a family member of the patient) has identical doubles or imposters; for example, a patient may believe that he has two wives, each of whom share nearly identical physical and personality characteristics, have the same number of children, have the same family background, etc.

- It is a relatively rare phenomenon and is far more disconcerting to the family than to the patient, who often seems unconcerned about these circumstances
- Although Capgras Syndrome can be the result of a psychiatric disturbance, up to 40% of patients with this disorder have been found to have organic brain disease
- Lesions in the Right Hemisphere, particularly those that disrupt frontoparietal pathways, are most often responsible
- There is no well-validated treatment

- Antipsychotic medications are not known to alter the Delusion
- Counseling family members that the patient's belief is the result of brain damage and does not represent negative feelings about them is suggested

Bouckoms, A., Martuza, R., & Henderson, M. (1986). Capgras syndrome with subarachnoid hemorrhage. *The Journal of Nervous and Mental Disease, 174*, 484–488.

Carotid Arteries. Two major arteries that supply blood to the brain; they enter the Circle of Willis and divide into the Anterior Cerebral Artery and the Middle Cerebral Artery, providing blood to Anterior brain structures; see Cerebral Circulation.

Category Test. A measure of Abstract Thinking, Problem Solving, and Conceptual Thinking sensitive to the presence of brain damage regardless of location; it is part of the Halstead-Reitan Neuropsychological Test Battery.

Caudate Nucleus. A Subcortical brain structure, part of the Basal Ganglia and the corpus striatum, involved in voluntary movement and possibly some cognitive functions such as language (on the left) and spatial Attention (in the Right Hemisphere); atrophy of the caudate has been associated with Huntington's Disease.

Central Sulcus. The large groove in the middle of each cerebral hemisphere that separates the Frontal Lobe from the Parietal Lobe; the convolution or gyrus that lies in front of (or Anterior to) the Central Sulcus is known as the Motor Strip or precentral gyrus and the gyrus that lies just behind (or Posterior to) to the Central Sulcus is known as the Sensory Strip or the postcentral gyrus.

Cerebellum. A brain structure that is positioned below the Cerebrum and behind the Brain Stem that controls motor coordination; it is composed of two hemispheres with each hemisphere controlling ipsilateral (same side) muscle coordination; a central portion of the Cerebellum, the vermis, controls midline structures such as the head, trunk, and neck; lesions to the Cerebellum can cause ipsilateral muscle incoordination (Ataxia) and intention tremors (tremors that occur when the patient moves willfully but are not present at rest); damage to the Cerebellum alone does not usually cause cognitive deficits.

Cerebral Circulation. The highly complex system of arteries and veins that supply blood (and oxygen, nutrients, etc.) to the brain.

- Although the brain accounts for only about 3% of body weight, it requires nearly 20% of the body's oxygen consumption
- Any disruption of blood flow to the brain from Cerebrovascular Accidents, Subarachnoid Hemorrhages, etc. can have significant effects upon cognitive functioning
- The major sources of blood supply to the brain are from the Carotid Arteries for the Anterior structures and the Basilar Artery for Posterior structures; see Figure 2 for further details (see also Circle of Willis).

Cerebrovascular Accident (CVA). CVAs or strokes result from the disruption of blood flow to the brain, which causes an alteration in the supply of oxygen and nutrients to brain structures.

- CVAs are the most common cause of neurologic disability in adults
- CVAs tend to produce focal and lateralizing damage that may include physical (e.g., hemipareis or hemiplegia), cognitive, and emotional alterations in the patient, some of which may be transient and others permanent and disabling
- The most important risk factor in stroke is advancing age; other important factors include hypertension, diabetes, elevated cholesterol levels, cardiac disease, family history, and smoking

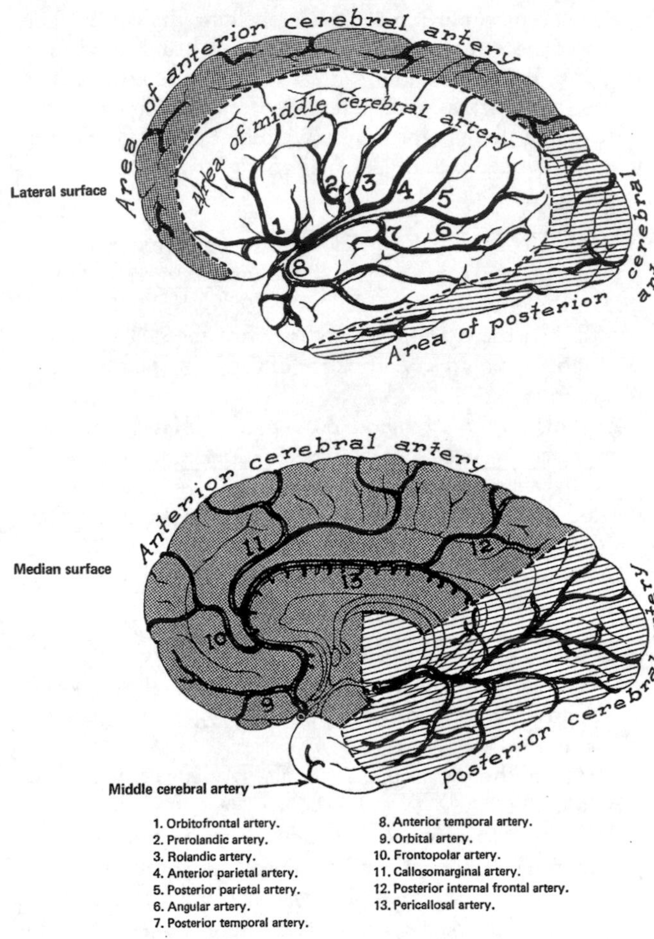

Figure 2. Scheme of the arterial supply of the cerebral cortex. (Reprinted, with permission, of author and publisher, from J. G. Chusid: *Correlative Neuroanatomy and Functional Neurology.* Appleton and Lange, 1982.)

- If stroke symptoms resolve within 24 hours the disorder is known as a Transient Ischemic Attack (TIA) and if the symptoms resolve within the first week the disorder is referred to as a Reversible Ischemic Neurologic Deficit (RIND)
- The two types of stroke are obstructive and hemorrhagic

Obstructive Cerebrovascular Accidents

- Obstructive strokes are the most common type of stroke
- They account for about 80% of all CVAs, and result in a blockage or an obstruction of blood flow to brain structures; this process is also known as Ischemia
- The disruption of blood flow creates an area of dead or damaged brain tissue known as an Infarct
- There are two types or causes of obstructive strokes
  - One is caused by the gradual narrowing of blood vessels by fat deposits, known as *thrombotic* strokes, which account for about 80% of obstructive CVAs
  - The other type of obstructive CVA is caused by the formation of a small particle elsewhere in the body which then travels to the brain and blocks a cerebral blood vessel (known as an embolus or an *embolic* stroke)
- The most common site for an obstructive stroke is in the distribution of the Middle Cerebral Artery

Hemorrhagic Cerebrovascular Accidents

- Hemorrhagic strokes account for about 20% of all CVAs
- Hemorrhages may result from Aneurysms, Artereovenous Malformations, and spontaneous bleeding from hypertension
- Acute survival rates tend to be lower for hemorrhagic than for obstructive strokes

Cognitive Deficits with CVAs

- Cognitive deficits following CVA depend on the location and size of the stroke as well as the patient's premorbid cognitive status
- During the acute recovery period, the patient's level of consciousness may be impaired and there may be evidence of global or diffuse cognitive impairments

- As the patient improves, more specific lateralizing signs will usually become apparent (e.g., left hemisphere strokes result in more language-based deficits and Right Hemisphere strokes cause more perceptual disorders)
- The cognitive effects of the stroke can be more disabling in patients with a prestroke history of Dementia and for patients with cortical Atrophy
- Some patients may present with multiple areas of ischemia in the White Matter of the brain; this may result in cognitive deficits with Memory and new learning, Concentration, and Mental Speed
- Multiple strokes can cause Dementia, known more specifically as multi-infarct or vascular Dementia

Emotional and Behavioral Deficits with CVAs

- Emotional and behavioral sequelae to stroke also depend on the location and size of the CVA
- Left hemisphere strokes tend to result in Depression and catastrophic reactions and Right Hemisphere strokes tend to result in indifference and poor Awareness of deficits
- In all, Depression is likely the most common Mood disorder following stroke and may occur in as many as half of all stroke survivors
- Other behavioral and emotional disorders may include irritability, Anxiety, Apathy, or Abulia, pathological laughing and crying (Pseudobulbar Affect), Agitation, and in rare cases, psychotic behavior
- An exaggeration of the patient's premorbid Personality characteristics or qualities is also not uncommon following CVA
- Referral to a stroke support group may be helpful for the patient and his or her family; contact the American Heart Association (214–373–6300)

Lezak, M. D. (1995). *Neuropsychological assessment* (3rd ed.). New York: Oxford University Press.

Cerebrospinal Fluid (CSF). A colorless fluid that flows through the Ventricles of the brain and in the Subarachnoid space outside the brain (see Arachnoid Layer); CSF is produced by the choroid plexus in the Ventricles and acts as a shock absorber for the soft tissues of the brain; an obstruction in the Ventricles or problems with reabsorption of the CSF can result in Hydrocephalus which can alter mental status; see also Intracranial Pressure.

Cerebrum. The most highly developed and organized brain structures that are most responsible for mediating cognition and behavior.

- It is composed of the left hemisphere (which is dominant for language-based functions in most people) and the Right Hemisphere (which is generally dominant for Perceptual Functioning)
- The hemispheres are connected by the Corpus Callosum
- The major subdivisions within the cerebral hemispheres include the Frontal Lobes, Temporal Lobes, Parietal Lobes, and Occipital Lobes
- The highest degree of specialization and localization of functions exists in the Cerebrum, although the Cerebrum works as an integrated whole with many brain areas contributing simultaneously to thinking and behavior; see Figure 3.

Children's Orientation and Amnesia Test (COAT). The children's equivalent of the Galveston Orientation and Amnesia Test (GOAT) for adults which assesses Orientation and Amnesia during acute recovery from Traumatic Brain Injury; serial administration of the COAT allows for objective and standardized assessment of Posttraumatic Amnesia (and its resolution) which is related to outcome; the COAT is for children ages 3–15 and consists of 17 questions in the areas of general Orientation (orientation to person and place, and recall of biographical information), temporal orientation, and Amnesia (immediate, recent, and associative Memory).

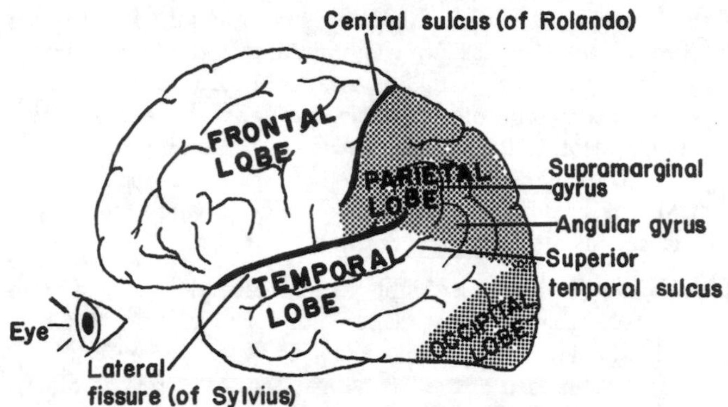

Figure 3. The cerebrum. (Reprinted with permission from *Clinical Neuroanatomy Made Ridiculously Simple* by Stanley Goldberg, 1997, p. 6. Miami, FL: Med Master.)

Ewing-Cobbs, L., Levin, H. S., Fletcher, J. M., Miner, M. E., & Eisenberg, H. M. (1990). The Children's Orientation and Amnesia Test: Relationship to severity of acute head injury and to recovery of memory. *Neurosurgery, 27*, 683–691.

Cingulate Gyrus. The Gyrus in each cerebral hemisphere that lies just above the Corpus Callosum which seems to exert subtle influence on Attention, intention, emotional expression, and Personality; reduced spontaneity and flattening of Affect can be sometimes observed in lesions to the Cingulate; bilateral damage to the Anterior portions of the Cingulate Gyrus can result in Akinetic Mutism.

Circle of Willis. Located at the base of the brain it provides the major arterial blood supply to the brain; it is formed from the junction of the internal Carotid Arteries and the Basilar Artery, both of which are its major sources of blood supply, and the Anterior Cerebral, Anterior Communicating, Posterior Cerebral, and Posterior Communicating Arteries; due to the many junctions and bifurcations of arteries in the Circle of Willis it is the most common site in the brain for Aneurysms; see Figure 4 (see also Cerebral Circulation).

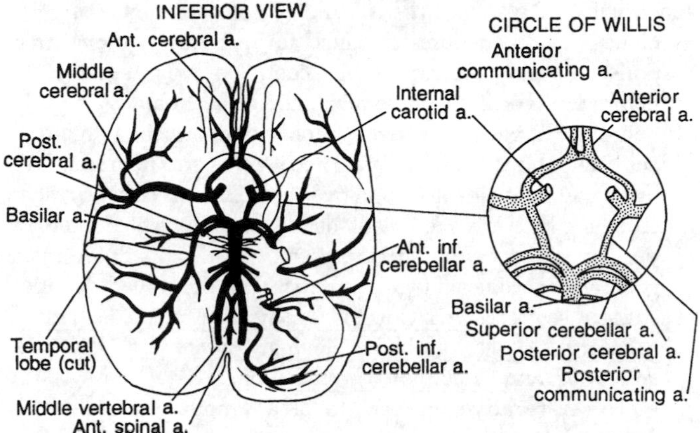

Figure 4. Major vascular supply of the cerebral cortex. (Reprinted with permission from *Anatomy and Physiology for Speech, Language, and Hearing* by J. A. Seikel, D. W. King, and D. G. Drumright, 1997, p. 469. San Diego: Singular Publishing Group.)

Circumlocution. A lack of precision in expressive language whereby the individual is unable to get to the point or "talks around" a topic or word; may be due to Anomia or other language problems or difficulty with thought organization.

Clock Drawing. A frequently used screening measure in neuropsychology in which the person is asked to draw the face of a clock and set the hands to a specific time, such as "10 after 11"; it can be sensitive to perceptual problems such as left Neglect (if the numbers do not extend to the left-hand side of the clock), poor organization (numbers are poorly spaced), or Concrete Thinking (the hands of the clock are set to the 10 and the 11).

Cochlear Nerve. One of two divisions of the Acoustic Nerve (Cranial Nerve VIII) which transmits auditory impulses from the ear to the cerebral hemispheres; damage to the Cochlear Nerve can cause hearing loss or Tinnitus.

Cognitive Rehabilitation. A set of interventions, techniques, and procedures designed to improve cognitive functions following damage to the central nervous system; the manner in which cognitive rehabilitation techniques affect the neurological basis of recovery is unknown (much is unknown generally about how the brain recovers at the neuronal level from trauma or insult); cognitive rehabilitation (CR) is still an emerging field in which many decisions about which interventions work best with specific cognitive deficits still are made generally by clinical judgment rather than by proven empirical studies; see also Behavior Management, Arousal, Attention, Memory, Abulia, Problem Solving, Awareness, Executive Functions, and Perceptional Functioning.

- The **restorative** approach to CR attempts to target the impaired area of functioning with a series of selectively challenging tasks or activities designed to *restore* or "cure" the deficit
  - This approach may have some utility in the treatment of more basic or fundamental abilities such as Attention, Concentration, and Mental Speed or reaction time although its impact on functional skills may be limited (an example of this approach would be to expose the patient with an attentional deficit to a series of challenging attention tasks on a computer)
  - A problem with this approach is the lack of generalizability between the tasks performed in therapy and the expression of the skill in daily life
  - These techniques are ineffective in resolving severe Memory disorders or Amnesia
- Another major intervention in CR is the **compensatory** approach in which the objective is focused toward facilitating return of functional activities of everyday life by helping the patient compensate or substitute an impaired function for a more intact ability
  - This approach helps patients to anticipate how their deficit may affect their functioning and to develop strategies to

compensate for them (an example would be using a Memory Log to help with a Memory impairment, rather than attempting to improve Memory functioning itself)
- Compensatory approaches have generally received greater acceptance in rehabilitation than have restorative ones
- Compensatory interventions require adequate Awareness of deficits on the patient's part in order to be effective (otherwise the patient will not use the strategies)

- A **holistic** or multimodal approach to CR can include the strategies described before but also underscores the need to consider other noncognitive variables in restoring functional capabilities in patients; these variables may include the patient's emotional status, social and cultural issues, self-concept, Awareness, and metacognition (a person's thinking about his or her thinking)

Suggestions for Establishing a CR Plan

- Establish the areas of deficit
- Carefully observe the patient's functioning to determine which specific activities are most problematic
- Give patients enough freedom to first complete the task unsuccessfully (do they know the task is not performed properly?) and then provide cues in a hierarchical fashion to determine what kind of help is beneficial
- Ask patients what they are thinking as they are attempting to perform an activity (i.e., do they know what to do next but can't quite figure out how, do they not know what they should be doing in the activity, what variable are they considering when performing the task?)
- Neuropsychological evaluation should be conducted to more objectively define the underlying deficit that may be interfering with daily living skills
- Determine through the previous assessments not only the patients' weaknesses but also their strengths which can be used to help them compensate for areas of impairment
- Establish the premorbid level of functioning of the patient

  - Determine premorbid cognitive strengths and weaknesses, particularly in the elderly where there may be a question of an underlying Dementia or in cases where the patient has low occupational or educational attainment
  - The patient's socioeconomic status may affect what types of CR activities he or she may be willing to engage in (e.g., patients who are a bit more "intellectual" will likely respond more favorably to a more scientific or didactic approach than patients with lower levels of education)
- Assess the premorbid coping strategies and Personality of the patient as this will provide some information about his or her response to direction, a willingness to confront problems, relationship with family members, the need to be in control or dependent on others, etc.
- Establish the CR goals
  - CR plans work best when they are focused; do not try to do too much at one time
  - Focus on those cognitive problems that are interfering most with progress in rehabilitation and for which improvement can be expected
  - CR goals should also be established by considering the most elementary or fundamental skills that need improving before higher level or more complex activities can become the focus of treatment
  - An estimation of the patient's recovery (rate, types of persistent deficits expected, etc.) based on injury parameters, neuroimaging results, time since injury, etc. should be considered in establishing CR goals and interventions (some prediction of recovery is necessary in order to determine which abilities are most likely to improve and within what time frame)
  - Establish goals that are as concrete and measurable as possible
  - The goals and plans should be established by the whole team, not dictated by only one person

- Try to include goals that will also be important to the patient although if insight is decreased the patient may minimize or deny all problem areas
- Take the time to establish the goals and the interventions; do not rush the process
- Assess the patient's current emotional status to determine how to approach the patient psychologically with the CR plan and interventions
- Awareness and insight into deficits, their affect on functional skills, and the need for rehabilitation are crucial factors in the CR process and must be addressed in the CR plan
- Review the CR plan with patients, why it is important, the expected outcome, and how it will affect their daily functioning
- Educate and include family members in the CR plan as much as possible; encourage them to review the goals and interventions with the patient; support them in interacting with the patient in a way that has been suggested by the CR plan
- Give continual and concrete feedback to patients about their performance during therapy and how it relates to the CR plan; be positive; praise even small gains and effort
- All treating therapists need to be involved in the CR plan and everyone working with the patient needs to understand what the interventions are; if specific tasks need to be done, they should be assigned to specific individuals (e.g., the speech therapist will put the Orientation information on the patient's bulletin board)
- CR is labor intensive; special time may need to be allocated to discuss patients and to establish CR activities as these issues may require more time than what is available during general team conferences

Guilmette, T. J., & Kennedy, M. L. (1995). Neurocognitive rehabilitation guidelines for therapists. *Topics in Stroke Rehabilitation, 2*, 32–43.

Coma. A state of unconsciousness in which the individual responds minimally or not at all to external stimuli and initiates no voluntary activities; it typically results from damage to the Reticular Activating System or to dysfunction in both cerebral hemispheres caused by trauma, Tumors, Cerebrovascular Accidents, or metabolic abnormalities; coma should be distinguished from other disorders of Arousal in which the patient may be lethargic or stuporous; coma should also be distinguished from Akinetic Mutism and Locked-in Syndrome; in true coma, there are no sleep-wake cycles and the eyes remain closed; see also Coma Vigil.

Coma in Traumatic Brain Injury

- Length of coma or unconsciousness is one of three indices of injury severity in Traumatic Brain Injury (the other two are length of Posttraumatic Amnesia and admitting Glasgow Coma Scale score)
- A person may sustain a brain injury without being in a coma or losing consciousness
- A person may become comatose without direct trauma to the head or skull (a "whiplash" effect in which the head is rapidly moved forward and backward can result in damage to the Axons which can render a person unconscious)
- Coma may occur immediately at the time of trauma, which is usually the case with Diffuse Axonal Injury, or may occur later as a result of brain swelling, Hemorrhage, Hydrocephalus, etc.
- The most widely used measure of depth of coma is the Glasgow Coma Scale (GCS), which is based on the patient's best motor, verbal, and eye opening response; the GCS has a range of scores from 3 (worst) to 15 (best; alert and oriented)
  - GCS score 13–15 = Mild Traumatic Brain Injury
  - GCS score 9–12 = moderate Traumatic Brain Injury
  - GCS score 3–8 = severe Traumatic Brain Injury
- Length of coma is also used to categorize severity of brain injury

- Mild Traumatic Brain Injury: 30 minutes or less of coma (if at all)
- Moderate Traumatic Brain Injury: greater than 30 minutes but less than 6 hours (the cutoff between moderate and severe TBI is not well defined; some may argue that up to 24 hours of coma would still consitute a moderate TBI)
- Severe Traumatic Brain Injury: greater than 6 hours (or perhaps greater than 24 hours)

- The longer the length of coma the worse the outcome generally although the relationship is far from perfect (i.e., some persons with shorter lengths of coma may have worse outcomes than other persons with longer comas)
- Coma 2 weeks or longer usually results in significant impairments and at least moderate disability—good outcomes are uncommon at this level
- In children, greater injury severity is necessary to produce a coma (i.e., children are more resistant to being rendered unconsciousness than adults)
- True coma (no Arousal, no Awareness, no sleep/wake cycles, eyes closed) usually lasts only 3 to 4 weeks and if consciousness is not obtained, it is followed by Coma Vigil or a vegetative state
- Patients evolve gradually out of coma and are disoriented and confused upon gaining consciousness
- Coma is always followed by a period of Posttraumatic Amnesia
- Agitation occurs following coma in about one third to one half of cases in TBI

Assessment of Coma

- There is no uniform measure for the assessment of low level patients (i.e., those patients still in or emerging from coma or a vegetative state); a sample of instruments that have been used in rehabilitation to document depth of coma and recovery of low level or severely disabled patients includes

- Glasgow Coma Scale
- Disability Rating Scale
- Rancho Los Amigos Cognitive Scale (levels I–III)
- Western Neuro Sensory Stimulation Profile (WNNS)

Coma Stimulation

- Coma stimulation (CS) is a conceptual approach to treating patients in coma with environmental and sensory stimulation; there are no well controlled, empirical studies available to document the efficacy of CS in the recovery of patients in coma
- Environmental stimulation may include music playing in the room; talking to the patient; playing audiotapes of friends and family, the patient's favorite television programs or movies; and placing favorite objects, pictures, etc. around the room
- Sensory stimulation may include a more systematic intervention in which the patient is exposed to tactile (stroking, touching, the use of soft or rough fabrics, cool to warm water), olfactory (perfumes, foods, etc.), auditory (different sounds and voices), gustatory (different tastes, glycerin swabs, etc.), and vestibular stimulation (sitting patient up, use of tilt tables, etc.)

Furie, K., & Feldmann, E. (1994). Disorders of consciousness. In E. Feldmann (Ed.), *Current diagnosis in neurology* (pp. 308–312). St. Louis, MO: Mosby-Year Book, Inc.

Dikmen, S., & Machamer, J. E. (1995). Neurobehavioral outcomes and their determinants. *Journal of Head Trauma Rehabilitation, 10*, 74–86.

Katz, D. I. (1992). Neuropathology and neurobehavioral recovery from closed head injury. *Journal of Head Trauma Rehabilitation, 7*, 1–15.

Zasler, N. D., Kreutzer, J. S., & Taylor, D. (1991). Coma stimulation: A critical review. *NeuroRehabilitation, 1*, 33–40.

Coma Vigil. A state of unresponsiveness following brain injury; also referred to as a vegetative state in which the person's eyes are open (patients may orient visually to stimuli but do not track or sustain fixation on an object) and sleep/wake cycles are exhibited although there is no Awareness of or responsiveness to the environment and no purposeful behavior; this level of Coma is different from Akinetic Mutism and Locked-in Syndrome; recovery from the coma vigil state after Traumatic Brain Injury usually occurs within 6 months (recovery after 1 year is unusual, particularly for persons over the age of 40); the Thalamus appears to play a role in Awareness and in the vegetative state.

Kinney, H. C., Korein, J., Panigraphy, A., Dikkes, P., Goode, R. (1994). Neuropathological findings in the brain of Karen Ann Quinlan: The role of the thalamus in the persistent vegetative state. *New England Journal of Medicine, 330*, 1469–1475.

Levin, H. S., Saydjari, C., Eisenberg, H. M. et al. (1991). Vegetative state after closed-head injury: A traumatic coma data bank report. *Archives of Neurology, 48*, 580–585.

Zasler, N. D., Kreutzer, J. S., & Taylor, D. (1991). Coma stimulation: A critical review. *NeuroRehabilitation, 1*, 33–40.

Competence. The ability to understand the consequences and ramifications of one's decisions; competence is usually related to a specific area (e.g., competence to make health care decisions, competence to handle one's finances, etc.) rather than a global determination (i.e., when assessing competence, the question becomes, "Competent to do what?"); patients must be aware of their disorder and its consequences in order to make competent decisions; competency may change over time and during treatment as patients' mental status improves.

Comprehension Subtest. A subtest on the Wechsler Adult Intelligence Scale—Revised and the Wechsler Intelligence Scale for Children—III which assesses common sense judgment and social intelligence.

Concentration. A basic or fundamental cognitive process for which there is no universally accepted definition but which is sometimes used interchangeably with Attention or, more specifically, with focused or selective Attention; may also refer to the ability to mentally manipulate information such as performing oral arithmetic, reciting digits backward (Digit Span), or naming the months of the year or days of the week in backward order.

- Some additional assessment measures of concentration include Trail Making Test, Stroop Color-Word Test, Paced Auditory Serial Addition Test, Controlled Oral Word Association Test, selected subtests from the Wechsler intelligence tests (Digit Span, Digit Symbol, Arithmetic), and the Attention/Concentration subtest of the Wechsler Memory Scale—Revised
- See the entry for Attention for examples of Cognitive Rehabilitation techniques

Conceptual Thinking. Refers to the quality or process of thinking in which the individual is able to think in useful generalizations (i.e., generalizing from a single instance), form abstract concepts, and apply procedural rules or principles to many situations; similar to Abstract Thinking; conceptual thinking is not linked to any one specific brain area, but rather is sensitive to the severity of brain trauma and to diffuse brain insults; an absence of conceptual functions results in Concrete Thinking; see Problem Solving for rehabilitation strategies.

- Some assessment measures for conceptual thinking include proverb interpretation, Category Test, Similarities, Comprehension, and Picture Arrangement subtests of the WAIS-R, Raven's Progressive Matrices, and the Wisconsin Card Sorting Test.

Lezak, M. D. (1995). *Neuropsychological assessment* (3rd ed.). New York: Oxford University Press.

Concussion. A generic term applied to the host of diverse symptoms following Mild Traumatic Brain Injury, including headache, dizziness, irritability, decreased Attention and Memory, and poor sleep.

Concrete Thinking. A sign of impaired or decreased Abstract and Conceptual Thinking which can affect efficient Problem Solving; can result from Aging Effects and from acquired brain injury; usually less apparent in individuals with higher levels of education.

Confabulation. A fabrication of recent events exhibited by some patients with Amnesia; the patient is unaware that his or her story is untrue; a way of "filling in the gaps" in a patient's recent Memory; it typically accompanies a lack of Awareness or Anosognosia for the Memory disorder and is more frequent during the early stages of recovery; most commonly reported with Korsakoff's Syndrome and with Frontal Lobe associated Memory disorders; should not be confused with a Delusion, which is usually fixed and unchanging over time (the confabulated story changes each time the patient is asked the same question, such as, "What did you do last night"); confabulations may be preposterous given the patient's circumstances and may respond only minimally to redirection.

Confusional State. A generic term used to describe the mental status of a patient who is alert but confused (not oriented and may be unaware of his or her surroundings), significantly inattentive, possibly inappropriate and irritable, and with significant Memory impairment; may be the result of metabolic encephalopathy, medication effects, or acute brain trauma/disease; during acute recovery from TBI, this would describe the patient in Posttraumatic Amnesia; in CVAs, acute confusional states tend to be more common in right than left hemisphere patients; see also Delirium.

Consciousness. An awake state; reflects the person's level of Arousal and alertness; sometimes used to refer to Awareness (of environment, others, the patient's disorder, etc.); usually presumes that the individual reacts or responds to the environment in some purposeful or meaningful manner; see Coma.

Constructional Ability. One of many Perceptual Functions that is particularly vulnerable to Right Hemisphere lesions (most notably Parietal Lobe dysfunction); it requires the ability to copy or reproduce by drawing or assembling blocks a visually presented model.

- The inability to copy visually presented stimuli is sometimes referred to as constructional Apraxia, although it is not likely a true Apraxia because the disorder is usually the result of perceptual problems and not motor programming
- Constructional impairment occurs more frequently than dressing Apraxia (approximately 4:1 ratio)
- In Right Hemisphere Cerebrovascular Accidents, constructional impairment is very common (it may occur between 35% to 90% in right CVAs) and is often accompanied by other visuoperceptual deficits such as unilateral spatial Neglect on drawings and Hemianopsia (the latter to a lesser degree); many other cognitive impairments can also be evident such as Anosognosia or decreased Awareness, and deficits with Attention, Impulsivity, and Problem Solving
- Constructional abilities have been shown to be associated with functional daily living skills such as dressing and meal preparation
- In addition to CVAs, constructional impairment can be evident with Traumatic Brain Injury, Dementia, chronic Alcohol use, or any brain insult that localizes to the right Parietal Lobe
- The most common assessment methods used for constructional abilities are simple drawing tasks (clock, Greek cross, daisy, house, etc.), complex drawings such as the Rey Osterrieth Complex Figure Drawing, and the Block Design subtest of the Wechsler intelligence tests

Treatment of Constructional Impairments

- Assess all aspects of cognitive and Perceptual Functions, particularly visual scanning, to determine the degree of underlying impairments that may affect constructional abilities (those underlying and accompanying deficits must also be addressed in therapy)
- Rule out problems with visual acuity, Hemianopsia, and motor function with the dominant hand (e. g., Apraxia, Ataxia)
- Have the patient *compare* two or more drawings for their similarities and differences
  - This will assess visual scanning and analysis without a motor component
  - If the patient is unable to do this type of activity accurately with even simple visual stimuli, then he or she would likely be unable to accurately draw designs
  - This technique could also be used as treatment
- Increase Awareness of perceptual problems and how they may affect the patient's functional skills (in Right Hemisphere patients, lack of insight is a common problem that can adversely affect treatment)
- Encourage patients to attend to and scan visual stimuli by systematically describing aloud the internal details and the external configuration before they attempt to draw or manipulate it (patients with Right Hemisphere syndromes may have more difficulty appreciating the external configuration of the design than the internal details)
- Establish a baseline of the type and complexity of designs that the patient is capable of copying
  - Systematically increase the complexity of the designs
  - Ask the patient to evaluate his or her performance
  - Provide explicit feedback to the patient about his or her errors and correct reproductions
- If patients are unable to copy even simple designs, ask them to trace the design with a finger

- Encourage patients to use verbal strategies or "self-talk" when attempting a perceptual task and to "talk themselves through" the activity (e.g., "First I draw the straight line down, then it goes to the left, and then it goes up again.")
- Slow the patient down when performing constructional tasks and carefully monitor Impulsivity (patients with Right Hemisphere damage tend to be impulsive and inattentive); encourage the patient to approach all tasks in a deliberate and methodical manner
- Break perceptual tasks down into smaller, more manageable units which the patient can more easily integrate (this could be accomplished by drawing parts of designs in different color ink which the patient could systematically copy or by covering parts of the design while the patient draws it and then gradually uncovering the hidden parts as the patient completes more of the design)
- Use sticks or blocks to have the patient reproduce simple designs (rather than drawing it) as it may be easier for the patient to use a "trial and error" approach
- If the patient has a left Neglect, then place the design in the right, intact visual field (it can be moved gradually and systematically to the left as the patient learns to compensate for it)
- Assemble puzzles of appropriate complexity (again, have patients talk out loud about their strategy for assembling the pieces, what details they are attending to, and then discuss with them after the activity which strategies were more or less effective)
- Remind patients to use some of the strategies described before (e.g., analyzing visual stimuli prior to attempting a task, self-talk to guide behavior and strategies, completing part of the activity before systematically moving on to the next step) when approaching more functional activities such as grooming and dressing
- The carry-over or generalization from performing table-top constructional tasks to functional/everyday activities may be enhanced if the *process* or *method* of how the task should be approached is emphasized rather than the end result

- Patients with constructional impairments need to learn to approach activities slowly, deliberately, and systematically (regardless of outcome) given the likelihood of accompanying Impulsivity and poor Awareness of deficits, which can significantly affect safety and functional independence
- If these approaches to tasks are emphasized and reinforced during constructional excercises then they may carry over or generalize to other functional activities

Hier, D. B., Mondlock, J., & Caplan, L. R. (1983). Behavioral abnormalities after right hemisphere stroke. *Neurology, 33*, 337–344.

Neistsdt, M. E. (1993). The relationship between constructional and meal preparation skills. *Archives of Physical Medicine and Rehabilitation, 74*, 144–148.

Mori, E., & Yamadori, A. (1987). Acute confusional state and acute agitated delirium: Occurrence after infarction in the right middle cerebral artery territory. *Archives of Neurology, 44*, 1139–1143.

Continuous Performance Test (CPT). A generic term applied to measures of sustained Attention or vigilance in which stimuli (visual or auditory) are presented to a subject at a continuous rate (approximately one per second) over an extended period of time (in most cases 5 to 20 minutes); the subject is required to respond to a specific stimulus but not others; the task is intended to be dull and boring, which necessitates sustained Attention and impulse control on the part of the patient; CPTs are often used in the assessment of Attention Deficit Hyperactivity Disorder or in any disorder in which attentional problems are suspected; computer administrations are common; there are many versions of CPTs available on the market.

Contrecoup Injury. Traumatic injury to the brain that occurs on the opposite side from the site of the initial injury (the "coup") due to the rebound effect of the brain in the skull; in effect, the brain "bounces" from the site of the initial trauma to the opposite area of the skull, causing another site of injury.

Controlled Oral Word Association Test (COWAT). A measure of word fluency or production in which the subject is asked to produce as many words as possible beginning with a given letter in a limited period of time; the most common letters used are F, A, and S or C, F, and L; COWAT is sensitive to left hemisphere language disorders as well as to Frontal Lobe lesions; in younger children, producing words to a specific category, such as "foods," is used in place of letters.

Benton, A. L. (1969). Development of a multilingual aphasia battery: Progress and problems. *Journal of the Neurological Sciences, 9*, 39–48.

Benton, A. L., Hamsher, K. de S., & Sivan, A. B. (1994). *Multilingual Aphasia Examination*. Iowa City, IA: AJA Associates.

Strauss, E., & Spreen, O. (1991). A *compendium of neuropsychological tests: Administration, norms, and commentary*. New York: Oxford University Press.

Contusion (brain). A bruising, usually on the surface of the brain, from trauma to the head that causes minute bleeding but no other structural abnormality; in Traumatic Brain Injuries the most common sites for contusions are the Frontal Lobes and the Anterior portions of the Temporal Lobes due to the location of these structures in the skull.

Corpus Callosum. A large bundle of White Matter fibers that connects the cerebral hemispheres and that allows for interhemispheric communication; it forms the roof of the lateral and third Ventricles; the portions of the corpus callosum from Anterior to Posterior are referred to as the genu, trunk, and splenium, respectively

Cortex. The gray, convoluted outer layer of the brain composed of nerve cell bodies and their synaptic connections; it is the most highly organized and well developed brain system; necessary for the integration and modulation of complex behavior and thought.

Cortical Blindness. The inability to see due to bilateral damage to the visual cortex in the Occipital Lobes or to the the optic tracts; it may also be accompanied by Anton's Syndrome which is a denial of blindness.

Cranial Nerves (Cn). A group of 12 pairs of fiber tracts of the brain which originate in the Brain Stem and mediate several motor and sensory functions.

- **Cn I (Olfactory).** Controls the sense of smell.
- **Cn II (Optic).** Conveys visual information from the eye to the Cortex and light intensity from the eye to the Brain Stem.
- **Cn III (Oculomotor).** Controls pupillary constriction, upper eyelid elevation, and most eye movements.
- **Cn IV (Trochlear).** Controls downward and inward eye movements.
- **Cn V (Trigeminal).** Conveys sensation to the corneas, nasal and oral mucosa, and facial skin; also controls the muscles for chewing.
- **Cn VI (Abducens).** Controls lateral eye movements.
- **Cn VII (Facial).** Controls all facial muscles and for taste perception on the Anterior portion of the tongue.
- **Cn VIII (Acoustic).** One division of this nerve controls hearing and the other controls equilibrium, body position, and orientation to space.
- **Cn IX (Glossopharyngeal).** Controls swallowing and supplies sensation to the mucous membranes of the pharynx; also responsible for taste perception on the Posterior third of the tongue and for salivation.
- **Cn X (Vagus).** Controls swallowing, phonation, and movement of the uvula and soft palate.
- **Cn XI (Spinal Accessory).** Controls the sternocleidomastoid and the upper portion of the trapezius muscles.
- **Cn XII (Hypoglossal).** Controls normal tongue movements involved in swallowing and speech.

Craniopharyngioma. A calcified hypothalamic Tumor that occurs in both children and adults; it causes endocrine dysfunction and if large enough may cause visual field defects (from pressing on the optic chiasm) or Hydrocephalus (from compression of the third Ventricle).

Delirium. A disturbance of Attention and Awareness of the environment that results in a significantly reduced ability to focus and shift Attention.

- Delirium also results in a change in cognition (such as Memory impairment, disorientation, ability to follow commands, etc.) or a perceptual disturbance (such as Hallucinations or Illusions) that are not better accounted for by a preexisting or established Dementia
- The condition develops over a short period of time (hours to days) and tends to fluctuate during the course of the day (i.e., the patient may be more confused at night or in the morning)
- There may be a reversal of the day-night sleep-wake cycle
- There may also be rapid shifts of emotion or sustained emotional disturbances such as Depression or Anxiety
- There are many medical conditions that can create delirium including metabolic disorders, medication side effects, withdrawal from alcohol or other substances, cardiac conditions, etc.
- Acute recovery from Traumatic Brain Injury can create a delirium-like state although it is referred to as Posttraumatic Amnesia and is considered a normal phase of recovery for which there is no "medical" or pharmacologic cure
- Treating the underlying medical disorder is the primary intervention

Delusions. A fixed but false belief or idea about reality or oneself that is firmly held despite what almost everyone else believes and despite proof or evidence to the contrary.

- Delusions are common in psychiatric disorders, such as Schizophrenia, but can also occur in neurologic conditions, particularly with Right Hemisphere disorders and Dementia
- Examples of delusions in neurologic conditions include Capgras Syndrome, Reduplicative Paramnesias, and pathological jealousy (Othello Syndrome), although delusions about many other subjects can occur

- Delusions differ from Confabulation in that the latter does not remain fixed, but rather, may change from moment to moment
- Gently redirect patients with delusions to the correct reality, although rational arguments alone will not alter their beliefs
- Request that family members also help to gently challenge the patient's delusion as they will likely be more trusted by the patient than a staff member
- Minimize the attention paid to the delusion if possible, if it does not interfere with rehabilitation
- Referral to a psychiatrist or Neuropsychiatrist may be necessary.

Dementia. A general term used to describe the development of multiple cognitive impairments, but does not provide information about its etiology.

- Diagnostic criteria for dementia according to the Diagnostic and Statistical Manual of Mental Disorders (DSM) include (a) Memory impairment; (b) at least one other cognitive disturbance which may include Aphasia, Apraxia, or a disturbance in Executive Functioning; (c) the cognitive impairment must be severe enough to interfere in occupational or social functioning; (d) the cognitive impairment must represent a decline from prior levels of functioning; (e) the impairments cannot be due to a Delirium
- Historically, the term dementia referred to a progressive or irreversible course and many clinicians today likely still think of it in those terms, however, in the most current edition of DSM the definition of dementia is based on the pattern of cognitive deficits and carries no connotation about prognosis (thus it is technically possible to describe the effects of severe TBI as Dementia due to Head Trauma)
- Dementia, which is most prevalent in the elderly (see Aging Effects), can be due to Alzheimer's Disease, which is the most common type of dementia, or from many

other etiologies including multi-infarct or vascular causes (a series of small strokes which result in a step-wise but progressive deterioration in cognitive and physical functioning), Parkinson's Disease, Huntington's Disease, Multiple Sclerosis, brain Tumors, or Acquired Immunodeficiency Syndrome (AIDS)

- Patients may have a diagnosis of dementia prior to their CVAs or head injuries which may result in greater disability than with an isolated cerebral insult alone
- The diagnosis of dementia can sometimes be given erroneously and can be confused with normal aging; it is important to ask specific questions of the family about a patient's mental status prior to hospitalization, particularly with regard to the patient's short-term or recent Memory and ability to manage finances and household tasks
- Reversible causes for dementia, such as metabolic, endocrine, or nutritional disorders need to be ruled out before the diagnosis is given
- In the elderly, severe psychiatric disorders, particularly Depression, can produce dramatic changes in cognitive functioning that can mimic dementia
- Neuropsychological evaluations can be very important in the diagnostic assessment of dementia to establish an objective baseline of cognitive functioning (to compare with future evaluations to assess whether symptoms are progressive), to determine whether the patient's abilities are age-related, to determine if the pattern of impairments is consistent with a dementing disorder, depression, or normal aging, and to make recommendations regarding safety, competence, relative areas of strengths, etc.
- Dementia does not preclude a person's ability to participate in or benefit from rehabilitation although the treatment team will need to tailor the rehabilitation interventions to the patient's cognitive strengths and weaknesses
- See Alzheimer's Disease entry for specific treatment recommendations

Depression. A state of depressed mood (i.e., feeling down, blue, sad, pessimistic about the future, etc.) that may be accompanied by a loss of interest in usual activities, weight loss or gain, insomnia (particularly early morning awakening) or hypersomnia, fatigue or loss of energy, feelings of worthlessness, decreased Concentration or Memory, or suicidal thoughts; the patient should be referred for formal treatment which may include psychotherapy (counseling) and the use of antidepressant medications.

- Depression may be transient and mild or may substantially alter the patient's life and functioning
- It can be caused by a person's Adjustment to his or her disability or can be the direct result of organic factors from the injury to the brain (persons with damage to the left hemisphere seem more vulnerable to depression than with Right Hemisphere damage)
- Depression is the most common emotional problem following TBI and CVAs (one quarter to one half of patients will become significantly depressed) and can adversely affect a patient's participation in and outcome from rehabilitation
- A prior history of depression or substance abuse are risk factors for depression following brain injury
- Monitoring a patient's Mood and Adjustment to disability are important components of the rehabilitation process
- Depression is more common after the acute recovery period as patients become more aware of their limitations after they are home and have attempted to return (perhaps unsuccessfully) to their preinjury lifestyle
- Monitor Family Functioning as this will also affect a patient's mood (family members may also need to be treated)
- Patients with damage to the Frontal Lobes may *appear* to be depressed because of decreased drive or motivation although they deny feelings of sadness, pessimism, etc.; these patients require different treatment interventions

than those whose Mood is actually depressed; see Abulia, Executive Functioning, Frontal Lobes

- See Adjustment entry for treatment suggestions
- Refer the patient to a mental health professional (psychologist, psychiatrist, social worker, etc.) for a complete assessment and treatment if problems interfere with rehabilitation

Diagnostic and Statistical Manual of Mental Disorders (DSM). The official nomenclature of mental (i.e., emotional, psychological, behavioral) disorders; it contains diagnostic criteria and descriptions of several hundred psychiatric disorders; it is now in its fourth edition (DSM-IV) and was published in 1994 by the American Psychiatric Association.

Diaschisis. A depression of brain activity or of specific functions related to areas of the brain outside the immediate site of damage that occurs usually in cases of focal brain lesions; it is believed to be a temporary phenomenon that, as it resolves, allows the depressed functions to improve spontaneously.

Diffuse Axonal Injury (DAI). The generalized shearing and stretching of Axons resulting from rapid deacceleration injuries such as motor vehicle accidents or falls of greater than 6 feet.

- DAI is the most common pathology in Traumatic Brain Injury
- There is no direct measurement of or diagnostic marker for DAI (in severe cases, there may be evidence of scattered Hemorrhages in the deep White Matter, the Corpus Callosum, or the Midbrain; small amounts of Subarachnoid or intraventricular hemorrhages; diffuse swelling; or late onset cerebral Atrophy)
- DAI usually results in an immediate loss of consciousness without a lucid interval
- The severity of DAI may be estimated by the patient's clinical course, including immediate loss of consciousness,

length of unconsciousness, depth of Coma (see Glasgow Coma Scale), and length of Posttraumatic Amnesia
- Greater long-term neurobehavioral and cognitive deficits are generally associated with more severe DAI

Bachman, D. L. (1994). Pain and trauma. In E. Feldman (Ed.), *Current diagnosis in neurology* (pp. 231–234). St. Louis, MO: Mosby-Year Book, Inc.

Katz, D. I. (1992). Neuropathology and neurobehavioral recovery from closed head injury. *Journal of Head Trauma Rehabilitation, 7,* 1–15.

Digit Span. The ability to repeat digits in forward order and in reverse order after they have been read aloud; digit span forward is a measure of Attention and immediate auditory Memory span (it is *not* a measure of short-term Memory); digit span backward also measures Attention as well as Concentration and perhaps "working Memory"; reversing digits is a more complex mental activity and is likely somewhat more sensitive to brain dysfunction than is repeating digits forward; there is usually only a difference of 1 or 2 digits between the forward and backward span in a non-brain-injured population; it is also a subtest on the Wechsler Intelligence Scale for Children—III and the Wechsler Adult Intelligence Scale—Revised.

Digit Symbol. A subtest on the Wechsler Adult Intelligence Scale—Revised and on the Wechsler Intelligence Scale for Children—III (where it is called Coding) which requires the person to transcribe geometric symbols that are matched with a particular number onto an answer sheet on which only the numbers are written, within a specified time period; this subtest measures motor speed and Attention; it appears to be one of the most sensitive subtests on the Wechsler Intelligence Tests to brain injury and is particularly sensitive to the effects of TBI in children.

Diplopia. Double vision; when caused by neurologic injuries it will usually be present only in certain directions of gaze and will not be present when one eye is covered; its most common causes are Brain Stem Infarct or injuries to Cranial Nerve III (Occulomotor) or VI (Abducens).

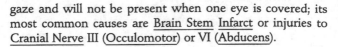

Disinhibition. The inability to inhibit or "hold back" impulsive responses, particularly in a social context; examples include swearing, telling inappropriate jokes, violating social rules/norms in conversations, inappropriate touching of self or others, etc.; disinhibition can cause significant social and vocational disability, and result in substantial social isolation for the patient and the family; associated with damage, often from TBI, to the orbitomedial portions of the Frontal Lobes; see also Executive Functions.

Treatment of Disinhibition

- Conduct comprehensive assessment to understand patient's cognitive strengths and weaknesses which will need to be incorporated into the patient's treatment team
- Obtain background information on the patient's premorbid emotional and social functioning
- Remain hopeful and optimistic with patient that behaviors can be changed and modified
- See Behavior Management entry for techniques to reward/reinforce appropriate behavior and extinguish inappropriate responses
- Increase patients' Awareness and insight into how their behavior affects others
- Educate patients about the effects of their injury on their social functioning
- Give patients specific and concrete feedback about their interpersonal behavior and alternative ways of responding
- Use Social Skills Training to alter and teach new interpersonal behaviors
- Use group formats to give patients feedback about their behavior, to practice new interpersonal skills, and to receive support from others with similar problems
- Help patients anticipate social situations that may cause difficulty and how they can best respond

- Educate family about social disability associated with TBI and their role in the treatment of this problem
- Psychotherapy or counseling may be helpful to assist patients in increasing their social sensitivity, adjusting to their altered functioning, and in remaining invested in treatment

Disability Rating Scale (DRS). An objective scale designed to monitor recovery from severe brain injury, which consists of the following eight items and score ranges: eye opening (0–3); verbal response (0–4); motor response (0–4); cognitive ability in feeding (0–3); cognitive ability in toileting (0–3); cognitive ability in grooming (0–3); dependence on others (0–5); employability (0–3); the scores from each of the eight items are summed with a lower score denoting less disability (0 = no disability) and a higher score reflecting greater disability; DRS has been shown to be more sensitive than the Glasgow Outcome Scale in following recovery from TBI and that higher scores are associated with longer lengths of stay in rehabilitation hospitals.

Eliason, M. R., & Topp, B. W. (1984). Predictive validity of Rappaport's Disability Scale in subjects with acute brain dysfunction. *Physical Therapy, 64*, 1357–1360.

Hall, K., Cope, D. N., & Rappaport, M. (1985). Glasgow Outcome Scale and Disability Rating Scale: Comparative usefulness in following recovery in traumatic head injury. *Archives of Physical Medicine and Rehabilitation, 66,* 35–37.

Rappaport, M., Hall, K. M., Hopkins, K., Belleza, T., & Cope, D. N. (1982). Disability Rating Scale for severe head trauma: Coma to community. *Archives of Physical Medicine and Rehabilitation, 63*, 118–123.

Doll's Eye Maneuver. Also known as the oculocephalic reflex, this maneuver is used in the comatose patient to assess the neural pathways from the Brain Stem controlling eye movements; if the head is rotated in one direction, the eyes should deviate together in the opposite direction (e.g., if the head is rotated to the right, the eyes should initially deviate to the left); if the eyes do not deviate then the Brain Stem may be injured.

Dura Mater. The outermost and most fibrous of the three membranes that cover the brain and spinal cord; see Meninges, Subdural.

Dysarthria. A disorder of articulation and the motor/muscular control of speech.

Dysphagia. Disorders of swallowing.

Dyslexia. A developmental reading disability; in the general population dyslexia is often thought to describe the problem of "reading" words or letters backward although this is only one, minor type of reading problem; most dyslexias are due to a person's inability to accurately translate graphemes (letters or letter combinations) into phonemes (sounds); persons with dyslexia are almost always poor spellers although the converse is not necessarily true; dyslexia is not related to Intelligence although other language based Learning Disabilities can accompany this problem.

Echolalia. The repetition of words or phrases (parrotted speech) made by others; may be evident in certain types of Aphasia and some developmental disorders such as autism.

Echopraxia. The automatic mimicking of others' movements; may be associated with tic disorders or Frontal Lobe syndromes.

Ecological Validity. The ability of a test to predict or measure "real world" functions such as the ability to live independently, work, handle one's finances, drive, etc.

Sbordone, R. J., & Long, C. J. (Eds.). (1996). *Ecological validity of neuropsychological testing.* Delray Beach, FL: GR Press/St. Lucie Press.

Electroencephalogram (EEG). An instrument used to measure the electrical activity of the Cortex through electrodes placed on specific areas of the scalp; helpful in the assessment of Seizures and in determining brain activity (brain waves) following brain injury; in most cases the EEG does not definitively rule in or rule out seizures as many persons with seizures have normal EEGs and some persons without seizures may have nonspecific EEG changes.

Embolism. A clot or plug that is formed elsewhere in the body, such as the heart, and travels via the circulatory system to a blood vessel of smaller size, causing a blockage of blood flow through that artery; a frequent cause of Cerebrovascular Accidents and Infarcts.

Encephalitis. An inflammation of the brain that can be caused by infection from virus, bacteria, parasites, etc.; see Herpes Simplex Encephalitis.

Encephalopathy. A nonspecific term used to describe any disease or disorder of the brain.

Epidural Hematoma. A large, rapidly expanding Hematoma that develops between the inner surface of the skull and the outer surface of the Dura Mater, usually from a laceration to the middle meningeal artery as a result of temporal bone fractures in TBI; its rate of expansion quickly produces Mass Effect and death unless immediate surgery is able to stop the bleeding.

Epilepsy. See Seizures.

Executive Functions. A term used to describe a broad set of abilities necessary for independent, appropriate, and self-serving behaviors that are frequently disrupted following TBI; these functions are typically associated with the Frontal Lobes but also likely encompass a broad set of brain regions; executive functions involve *how* things get done (e.g., the planning, organization, direction, and control of behavior) not just what gets done; these abilities are crucial for independent functioning in the home, community, and at work or school.

- There is no cohesive or highly specific definition for executive functions although several authors have proposed conceptual models for disorders of this type
- Lezak (1995) suggested that executive functions include the following abilities:
  - *Volition:* Refers to the capacity for intentional behaviors; requires Motivation and the capacity for self-Awareness
  - *Planning:* The identification and organization of the steps necessary to carry out an intention or achieve a goal
  - *Purposive Action:* The translation of an intention or plan into productive, self-serving activity; requires the ability to initiate, maintain, switch, and stop sequences of complex behavior; involves the regulation of behavior—the ability to be productive, to be flexible, and shift behavior or Problem Solving strategies as necessary (Perseveration would be an outcome if this ability were deficient)
  - *Effective Performance:* Requires the ability to monitor, self-correct, and regulate the intensity, tempo, and other qualitative aspects of one's behavior or Problem Solving; to perceive, identify, and correct errors as necessary with one's performance

- Stuss and Benson (1986) proposed a hierarchy of three levels of brain functions related to frontal and executive abilities that include drive and sequencing at one level; anticipation, goal-selection, preplanning, and monitoring on the next; and self-awareness at the highest level

Assessment of Executive Functions

- Due to the complexity and variability of executive functions, there is no one test or test battery that has been proven to provide a specific measurement of abilities in this area
- Executive function deficits can exist with intact Intelligence, Memory and other cognitive skills
- Some neuropsychological tests that may provide a partial analysis of executive functions include the Category Test, Wisconsin Card Sorting Test, Controlled Oral Word Association Test, Porteus Mazes, Trail Making Test, Rey-Osterrieth Complex Figure, Design Fluency Test, Stroop Color-Word Test, Tinker Toy Test, copying of repeated patterns or designs, Cancellation Tests, and measures of motor programming, speed, and coordination
- Formal tests of cognitive functioning are often too structured to provide a comprehensive assessment of executive skills
- Establish patients' preinjury Personality (is it now changed and in what manner?), their ability to get along with others, and their social sensitivity
- Establish patients' preinjury ability to be productive, follow through on tasks, plan and organize themselves, and remain motivated and goal directed (there are many individuals who exhibit problems in these areas who have never had a neurologic injury so it is important to recognize which characteristics of the patient's behavior are acquired and which ones predated the injury)
- Observe patients as they try to solve "real life" problems or items on cognitive tests—how do they approach a task?—look for evidence of Impulsivity, poor planning,

Perseveration, poor initiation, disorganization in their approach to tasks, inability to shift Attention or Problem Solving strategies, and inaccurate self-appraisal of their own performance

- While observing patients' behavior during functional activities let them begin to fail (safely) the task and observe if they notice their problems and how they may try to correct them
- Discuss with the patient's family members their observations of the patient's behavior and ability to initiate, plan, organize, and follow through on goals and activities
- Evaluate cognitive functioning in multiple domains including Memory, Attention, language, Abstract Thinking, and Perceptual Functioning to assess relative strengths and weaknesses and to determine if other cognitive deficits could account for or contribute to limitations with executive functioning (for example, a patient with a Memory deficit may not complete or follow-through on tasks because he or she forgets what to do next and not because of inadequate drive, planning, etc.)
- Rule out or treat emotional and psychological factors such as Depression and Anxiety that could contribute to problems with executive functioning
- Integrate what is known about the patient's premorbid functioning with the results of the formal cognitive assessment, observations of the patient's behavior in treatment, and the family's report to determine which specific executive functions are deficient under which specific conditions or circumstances

Treatment of Executive Function Problems

- Treat problems with executive skills within the context of the Cognitive Rehabilitation plan and in conjunction with the treatment for other cognitive deficits
- The treatment plan must be individualized to accommodate patients' particular problems (strengths and weaknesses) and by respecting their psychosocial history and circumstances

- Educate the patient and the family about the role of executive functions in daily activities and the patient's specific strengths and weaknesses in this area
- Provide emotional support to the family and the patient during the recovery period
- Focus on promoting the patients' Awareness about their problems and their affects on daily functioning and on others
- See Abulia entry for treatment suggestions for problems with drive and initiation
- Give patients clear and specific expectations for their own daily care (e.g., the time they are to begin and finish dressing, prepare meals, and perform other household tasks)
- Have patients write out their daily schedules with the times they are to accomplish each task (and in which order), teach them to refer to it frequently, and check off each item/task as it is completed
- Use Behavior Management techniques to reinforce progress and effort toward appropriate behavior and to extinguish inappropriate behavior
- Deficits with planning and organization are addressed under the entry for Problem Solving
- See Social Skills Training for treatment suggestions for impaired social functioning
- Provide the necessary structure for the patient's daily routine with lists, schedules, reminders, etc. so that the patient is able to perform his or her daily activities successfully, then gradually and systematically reduce the amount of structure and support
- Use a wristwatch with a timer so that patients can be reminded when to refer to their schedule or to begin certain activities
- Ensure that patients know how to perform an activity before they are requested to perform it independently (e.g., make sure that the patient knows how to use the coffee pot before he or she is requested to make coffee as part of the AM routine)

- Assist the patient in determining which steps and in which order are necessary to complete specific tasks
- Instruct patients in how to monitor their performance and to ask themselves questions such as, "Am I completing this task accurately?"or "Is this how I had planned to do it?"

Cripe, L. I. (1996). The ecological validity of executive function tests. In R. J. Sbordone & C. J. Long (Eds.), *Ecological validity of neuropsychological testing* (pp. 171–202). Delray Beach, FL: GR Press/St. Lucie Press.

Lezak, M. D. (1995). Neuropsychological assessment (3rd ed.). New York: Oxford University Press.

Mayer, N. H., & Schwartz, M. F. (Eds.). (1993). Executive function disorders [Special issue]. *Journal of Head Trauma Rehabilitation, 8*(1).

Sohlberg, M. M., Mateer, C. A., & Stuss, D. T. (1993). Contemporary approaches to the management and control of executive control dysfunction. *Journal of Head Trauma Rehabilitation, 8,* 45–58.

Stuss, D. T., & Benson, F. D. (1986). *The frontal lobes.* New York: Raven Press.

Extinction. 1. Suppression of stimuli (tactile, visual, or auditory) on one side of the body, suggesting a lesion in the contralateral hemisphere, with bilateral simultaneous stimulation (e.g., lightly touching both hands simultaneously of the patient with his or her eyes closed but the patient being aware of only one hand being touched, or stimulating both visual fields simultaneously but the patient "seeing" only one side). 2. Eliminating a behavior by omitting reinforcement for it or by ignoring it; see Behavior Management.

Face Recognition. See Prosopognosia.

Facial Nerve. Cranial Nerve VII conveys taste sensation from the Anterior two thirds of the tongue and innervates the facial muscles for a person's frown, raised eyebrows, wink, smile, and grimace; the upper facial muscles are innervated by both cerebral hemispheres but the lower muscles are innervated by the contralateral hemisphere; the Facial Nerve originates in the Pons.

Facial Recognition Test. The Test of Facial Recognition was developed to assess a person's ability to recognize faces without a Memory component; in this test the subject is asked to match a picture of a person's face taken from various angles and with various lighting conditions from among six choices; it is sensitive to perceptual deficits and to Posterior brain lesions.

Benton, A. L., Hamsher, K. deS., Varney, N. R., & Spreen, O. (1983). *Contributions to neuropsychological assessment*. New York: Oxford University Press.

Family Assessment Device (FAD). A 60-item questionnaire designed to assess six specific dimensions of family functioning as well as an overall level of family functioning; the six dimensions include problem solving, communication, role dimension, affective responsiveness, affective involvement, and behavior control; the FAD has been used in several studies with neurologic patients and is available in a number of foreign languages.

Bishop, D. S., & Miller, I. W. (1988). Traumatic brain injury: Empirical family assessment techniques. *Journal of Head Trauma Rehabilitation, 3,* 16–30.

Epstein, N. B., Baldwin, L. M., & Bishop, D. S. (1983). The McMaster Family Assessment Device. *Journal of Marital and Family Therapy, 9,* 171–180.

Family Functioning. The premorbid functioning of families and their adjustment and adaptation to the patient's deficits can have significant ramifications for outcome in rehabilitation.

Family Functioning and Brain Injury

- The cognitive, personality, and behavior changes associated with brain injury are more difficult for families to deal with than are physical impairments
- Following Traumatic Brain Injury, families become most acutely aware of their loved one's level of disability in the second half of the first posttraumatic year (immediately after the trauma families' expectations for a full recovery are very high—optimism declines with time and experiences with the patient)
- Families assume a major portion of the care to survivors of TBI
- Disability resulting in job loss and increased need for medical/rehabilitative services can place a substantial financial burden on families, which creates increased stress
- Families can become socially isolated and the home may no longer be a "safe haven"; children and siblings may stop bringing friends home to socialize
- Depression is common in caregivers and in family members of persons with TBI and CVA
- Role reversals increase family tension (e.g., an injured spouse may become dependent and childlike; an adolescent may be required to look after his or her injured parent)
- Spouses may feel trapped and in "social limbo"; a loss of affection and sexual gratification in the marriage may occur
- A patient's lack of Awareness of his or her difficulties may increase family and marital conflict
- Some families can come through a crisis and function well

Suggestions for Improving Family Adaptation and Capabilities

- Consider the family as much as the patient in making treatment and discharge decisions
- Engage families as soon as possible
- Educate families about the rehabilitation process and the disorder of their loved one but recognize that too much information too early will likely be overwhelming

- Do not judge families due to differences in lifestyle or methods of communication
- Assess the functioning of the family via clinical interview and history taking; structured assessment instruments such as the Family Assessment Device may be particularly helpful
- The family must be informed and agree to any systematic Behavior Management program that is proposed for the patient
- Attend carefully to the physical and mental health (particularly Depression) of the caregivers (refer for treatment if appropriate)
- Focus on helping the family find the strengths in problematic, long-term relationships
- Ensure that the family's expectations for the patient's daily functional abilities are realistic and congruent with the team's expectations
- Help families to improve the capacity to solve problems, communicate, deal with change, and manage caregiving tasks
- Counseling may be necessary to improve family functioning
- Encourage (and provide if possible) support group attendance; investigate whether local chapters of the National Brain Injury Association offer support groups for TBI survivors and their families
- Provide specific and pragmatic help to families about how to manage the behavioral and emotional problems of the patient
- Normalize feelings of frustration, sorrow, and anger for family members of persons with brain injury
- Encourage caregivers to take care of themselves as much as their loved one
- Support caregivers to rely on their own conscience and judgment (and not everyone else's) in making decisions about their family member
- Ask family members what they need and how the rehabilitation team can help

Bishop, D. S., & Evans, R. L. (1995). Families and stroke: The clinical implications of research findings. *Topics in Stroke Rehabilitation, 2*, 20-31.

Lezak, M. D. (1978). Living with the characterologically altered brain injured patient. *Journal of Clinical Psychiatry, 39*, 592–598.

Lezak, M. D. (1986). Psychological implications of traumatic brain damage for the patient's family. *Rehabilitation Psychology, 31*, 241–250.

Tarvin, G. (1995). How to engage families in stroke rehabilitation. *Topics in Stroke Rehabilitation, 2*, 10–19.

Frontal Eye Fields. Located on the lateral portion of the Frontal Lobes and Anterior to the Motor Strip, the frontal eye fields contribute to ocular motility and are necessary for voluntary gaze and visual search; patients with lesions in the frontal eye fields cannot move their eyes to the contralateral side to command or when engaged in active visual searches but can passively move their eyes in that direction, demonstrating a lack of Neglect.

Frontal Lobes. The most Anterior and largest of the four lobes of the cerebral Cortex.

- Frontal Lobes are the most recent to develop in our species and are the last to fully mature in us as individuals (full maturation of the Frontal Lobes probably does not occur until early to middle adolescence)
- The Frontal Lobes contribute significantly to our uniqueness as a species and as individuals; they are responsible for complex brain-behavior relationships
- They are highly vulnerable to damage to the front of the head in TBI due their location and due to the proximity of boney protrusions inside the skull to frontal areas
- Blood supply to the Frontal Lobes occurs primarily via the Anterior Cerebral Artery and secondarily from the Middle Cerebral Artery; Aneurysms and Subarachnoid Hemorrhages in the area of the Anterior Communicating Artery can result in severe Frontal Lobe damage

- The Frontal Lobes have extensive connections with Posterior and Subcortical Structures (e.g., Thalamus and Basal Ganglia)
- Damage to the Frontal Lobes may result in significant Personality changes to the individual which may be the most disabling and the most difficult for family and friends to deal with
- Frontal Lobe damage can also result in changes to cognitive abilities (e.g., Memory, Attention, Problem Solving, etc.) and to a spectrum of complex, self-regulatory behaviors known as Executive Functions
- Major subdivisions of the Frontal Lobes and possible related neurobehavioral impairments include (see Figure 5):
  - *Posterior/Motor:* Hemiplegia on the contralateral side of the body, decreased strength or coordination
  - *Lateral:* Lesions to this area may result in poor ability to generate multiple Problem Solving strategies or response alternatives; failure to maintain Attention and "task set"; poor self-monitoring of errors; inability to shift Attention or ideas from one task to another; Perseveration; distractibility; poor organization and planning; inability to perform bilateral hand movements and alternating graphic sequences; nonfluent or Broca's Aphasia (left hemisphere); and left spatial Neglect (Right Hemisphere)
  - *Mesial:* Decreased drive and initiation (see Akinetic Mutism, Bradyphrenia, Abulia); inappropriate environmental searching (see Utilization Behavior and Alien Hand Syndrome)
  - *Orbital:* Anosmia; Amnesia with Confabulation; hypersensitivity to pain and noxious stimuli; Impulsivity; disihibited Personality and emotional responses; reduced empathy and self-awareness
- Assessment of Frontal Lobe functions requires a comprehensive neuropsychological evaluation to delineate the specific areas of cognitive strengths and deficits, careful observation of the manner in which the patient approaches tasks and responds to errors, attention to the patient's

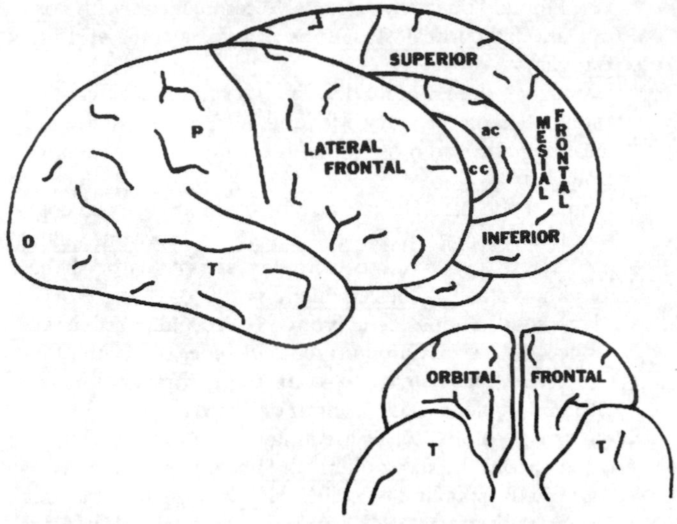

Figure 5. Regions of specialized functional-clinical significance include the lateral (also referred to as dorsolateral), superior mesial, inferior mesial and orbital sectors. (Abbreviations: O- *Occipital Lobe*, P-*Parietal Lobe*, T-*Temporal Lobe*, ac-*Anterior Cingulate*, (cc-*Corpus Callosum*). Schematic drawing of the frontal lobes of the brain. (Reprinted with permission from Impact of Frontal Lobe Lesions on Rehabilitation and Recovery from Acute Brain Injury by P. J. Eslinger, L. M. Grattan, and L. Geder, 1995, p. 163. *NeuroRehabiliation, 5*. Copyright Elsevier Science Ireland, Ltd.)

interpersonal and social behaviors, and information from the patient's family regarding behavioral and emotional functioning under less structured, "real world" conditions

Treatment of Frontal Lobe Disorders

- Due to the diversity and complexity of frontal behaviors, there is no single treatment plan or intervention that can address all possible neurobehavioral deficits

- Identify the 1 to 2 neurobehavioral impairments that interfere most with the patient's independent functioning
- Problems to address must be agreed on by the team and the patient's family
- An initial step of treatment must be to increase the patient's Awareness of the impairment (see Cognitive Rehabiliation) and to elicit some agreement with (or method to motivate the patient toward) the treatment goals
- Specific cognitive and neurobehavioral deficits can be addressed by referring to the following entries: Attention, Abulia, Agitation, Awareness, Executive Functions, Behavior Management, Social Skills Training, Problem Solving, Memory, and Impulsivity

Eslinger, P. J., Grattan, L. M., & Geder, L. (1995). Impact of frontal lobe lesions on rehabilitation and recovery from acute brain injury. *NeuroRehabilitation, 5*, 161–182.

Malloy, P., Bihrle, A., Duffy, J., & Cimino, C. (1993). The orbitomedial frontal syndrome. *Archives of Clinical Neuropsychology, 8,* 185–201.

Malloy, P., & Richardson, E. D. (1994). Assessment of frontal lobe functions. *Journal of Neuropsychiatry and Clinical Neurosciences, 6,* 399–410.

Stuss, D. T., & Gow, C. A. (1992). "Frontal dysfunction" after traumatic brain injury. *Neuropsychiatry, Neuropsychology, and Behavioral Neurology, 5,* 272–282.

Functional Disorder. A term historically used to describe a disorder or deficit due to a psychological or emotional cause rather than an organic one.

Functional Assessment Measure (FAM). An objective outcome measure designed specifically for use with persons who have sustained Traumatic Brain Injury which emphasizes the cognitive and psychosocial aspects of disability; it consists of 12 items (swallowing, car transfer, community mobility, reading, writing, speech intelligibility, emotional status, adjustment to limitations, employability, Orientation, Attention, and safety judgment) that are rated on a 7-point scale; the FAM items do not stand alone but are intended to be added to the 18 items of the Functional Independence Measure (FIM) to produce a 30-item scale combination referred to as the FIM+FAM; preliminary research suggests that the FAM may be more sensitive as a postacute than acute rehabilitation measure.

Hall, K. M., Hamilton, B. B., Gordon, W. A., & Zasler, N. D. (1993). Characteristics and comparisons of functional assessment indices: Disability Rating Scale, Functional Independence Measure, and Functional Assessment Measure. *Journal of Head Trauma Rehabilitation, 8*, 60–74.

Functional Independence Measure (FIM). An objective measure of independent functioning, developed by a national rehabilitation task force, that is used to monitor recovery and outcome in rehabilitation; it consists of 18 areas of functioning including ambulation, self-care, communication, and cognitive skills, each rated on a scale of 1 (fully dependent) to 7 (fully independent); the FIM was also developed to be a national standard of disability assessment, to be discipline free, and to represent a minimal data set to compute the cost and efficacy of rehabilitation; see also Functional Assessment Measure.

Hall, K. M., Hamilton, B. B., Gordon, W. A., & Zasler, N. D. (1993). Characteristics and comparisons of functional assessment indices: Disability Rating Scale, Functional Independence Measure, and Functional Assessment Measure. *Journal of Head Trauma Rehabilitation, 8*, 60–74.

Galveston Orientation and Amnesia Test (GOAT). A standardized test of Amnesia and Orientation used to evaluate recovery from Posttraumatic Amnesia following Traumatic Brain Injury; it is based on a scoring system of 0–100; a score of >75 on two consecutive days is associated with resolution of Posttraumatic Amnesia.

Levin, H. S., O'Donnell, V. M., & Grossman, R. G. (1979). The Galveston orientation and amnesia test: A practical guide to assess cognition after head injury. *Journal of Nervous and Mental Diseases, 167,* 675–684.

Gerstmann's Syndrome. A constellation of four symptoms that include finger Agnosia, right/left disorientation, Acalculia, and Agraphia associated with lesions in the dominant Parietal Lobe or at the parietal-occipital junction; there is some controversy about whether there is a relationship among these four findings and whether they consistently localize to the same brain area.

Glasgow Coma Scale (GCS). A practical and reliable assessment procedure to evaluate depth of Coma based on three components of wakefulness in the patient (i.e., the stimulus needed to induce eye opening, the best motor response, the best verbal response); the range of GCS scores is 3–15; initial GCS scores are important indicators of the severity of Traumatic Brain Injury and are helpful in predicting long-term outcome along with length of Coma and length of Posttraumatic Amnesia; severity of TBI is associated with the following GCS scores: mild TBI = 13–15; moderate TBI = 9–12; severe TBI = 8 or less.

Scoring of the Glasgow Coma Scale

Eyes opening	*Score*
Never	1
To pain	2
To sound/verbal stimuli	3
Spontaneously	4

Best verbal response	
None	1
Incomprehensible sounds	2
Inappropriate words	3
Disoriented but converses	4
Oriented and converses	5
Best motor response	
None	1
Extension (decerebrate response)	2
Abnormal flexion (decorticate response)	3
Flexion withdrawal	4
Patient localizes to pain	5
Patient obeys commands	6
Total	3–15

Teasdale, G., & Jennett, B. (1974). Assessment of coma and impaired consciousness: A practical scale. *Lancet, 2*, 81–84.

Glasgow Outcome Scale (GOS). A scale used to categorize outcome in TBI based on a patient's physical and economic dependence and social reintegration; the scale uses four levels of recovery: persistent vegetative state, severe disability, moderate disability, and good recovery; because only four levels of recovery are described, the moderate category likely encompasses a wide range of outcomes and may not accurately reflect the abilities or impairments of patients who fall at the extremes of that level.

Jennett, B., & Bond, M. (1975). Assessment of outcome after severe brain damage. *Lancet, 1,* 480–487.

Glioblastoma. A highly malignant and infiltrating brain Tumor that occurs mostly in adults; it typically develops in the Cerebrum and grows rapidly; it is a type of Astrocytoma.

Glioma. A type of brain Tumor that results from malignant transformation of glial cells which are the cells that form the connective tissue in the central nervous system; glial tumors consist mostly of astrocytes (which include Astrocytomas and Glioblastomas) and oligodendrogliomas.

Glossopharyngeal Nerve. Cranial Nerve IX is one of the four bulbar Cranial Nerves (so named because they originate near the Medulla which was once called "the bulb"); it controls swallowing and supplies sensation to the mucous membranes of the pharynx as well as providing taste perception to the Posterior third of the tongue and for salivation.

Guillain-Barré Syndrome (GBS). An acute inflammatory or postinfectious polyneuropathy that initially presents with numbness and parathesias in the fingers and toes but which can ascend to total paralysis requiring intubation for respiratory support; GBS itself does not result in cognitive deficits although secondary complications from Anoxia and medication side effects can alter mental status; patients who have required intubation may also develop high levels of Anxiety during their recovery with fears of suffocation, the return of the illness, and being left alone.

Gyrus. The convolutions in the Cerebrum that lay between the grooves or sulci.

Hallucination. A sensory perception that the patient believes to be real but occurs without actual external stimulation; the most common hallucinations are visual (seeing objects, people, images that are not there), auditory (hearing sounds or voices that are not there), gustatory (perceiving tastes that are not present), and Olfactory (perceiving odors that are not pleasant); see Illusion.

- In psychiatric disorders, hallucinations are associated with severe mental illness such as Schizophrenia
- Patients with neurologic disorders may have hallucinations without any history of mental illness
- In neurologic disorders, hallucinations are more common with lesions to the Right Hemisphere than the left hemisphere; Right Hemisphere damage tends to produce visual hallucinations and left hemisphere damage tends to produce auditory hallucinations
- Following a brain insult, hallucinations tend to occur more during the acute recovery period than later in recovery
- Hallucinations are common during a Delirium or Acute Confusional State
- Seizures may cause hallucinations, particularly Olfactory and gustatory

Halstead-Reitan Neuropsychological Test Battery. A structured neuropsychological test battery composed of the following tests: Category Test, Finger Oscillation Test, Seashore Rhythm Test, Tactual Performance Test, and Speech Sounds Perception Test; the battery produces an Impairment Index that reflects the number of tests that fall in the "brain damaged" range.

Hematoma. A collection or accumulation of blood that may occur rapidly or slowly, usually from a Traumatic Brain Injury but may also occur from spontaneous bleeding due to hypertension or other factors; hematomas may be Subdural, Intracerebral, or Epidural.

Hemianopsia. A Visual Field Cut that produces blindness in one half of the visual field; it is the result of a disruption of the optic fibers that carry visual signals from the brain to the calcarine cortex of the Occipital Lobes; it is not the result of problems with the eye itself and is not the same as a Neglect (hemianopsia can be compensated for much easier than a Neglect, which is a deficit of spatial Attention); the most common cause is Cerebrovascular Accidents.

Hemorrhage. Bleeding; it most often occurs from trauma, hypertension, or a ruptured Aneurysm; the most common areas for hemorrhage within the brain are in the Subarachnoid space, Subdural space, Epidural space, within the Ventricles (intraventricular) or within the gray/White Matter of the Cerebrum (Intracerebral).

Herniation. A protrusion or displacement of brain structures from a mass lesion or diffuse swelling; the herniation often occurs with a downward displacement or swelling of the Temporal Lobe, resulting in a decreased level of consciousness, dilatation, and loss of light reactivity of the ipsilateral pupil due to compression of Cranial Nerve III, and hemiparesis on the contralateral side; compression of the Midbrain and Pons may also occur which may result in Brain Stem failure (e.g., respiratory abnormalities, changes in heart rate and respiration); see Mass Effect and Midline Shift.

Herpes Simplex Encephalitis. The most common, nonepidemic viral Encephalitis that can result in severe cognitive impairments; the Herpes Simplex virus has a predilection for gravitating toward the undersurface of the Frontal and Temporal Lobes which can cause dramatic Memory deficits, Personality changes, and Seizures.

Hippocampus. Bilateral Subcortical Structures that lie on the medial (inner) surface of the Temporal Lobes believed to be critical for short term Memory; sensitive to the effects of Anoxia.

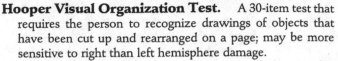

Hooper Visual Organization Test. A 30-item test that requires the person to recognize drawings of objects that have been cut up and rearranged on a page; may be more sensitive to right than left hemisphere damage.

Hooper, H. E. (1983). *Hooper Visual Organization Test.* Los Angeles: Western Psychological Services.

Huntington's Disease. An inherited progressive illness characterized by chorea (random jerking movements of the body) and Dementia; onset is typically in middle age and becomes fatal within 10 to 20 years; the Dementia often occurs soon after the physical manifestations of the disease and can be accompanied by changes in Personality.

Hydrocephalus. An abnormal accumulation of Cerebrospinal Fluid (CSF) in the cranial vault that may be developmental or acquired; see also Normal Pressure Hydrocephalus.

- Communicating hydrocephalus occurs when the CSF flows unobstructed through the Ventricles but is not reabsorbed fast enough; thus, the brain is producing more CSF than it can absorb
- Noncommunicating or obstructive hydrocephalus occurs when the passage of CSF through the Ventricles is blocked
- Hydrocephalus *ex vacuo* occurs when the amount of CSF and Ventricles expand to replace brain tissue lost from Atrophy
- Hydrocephalus causes increased Intracranial Pressure which results in Ischemia and possible compression of important brain structures
- Hydrocephalus may develop after brain injury and may require that a Shunt be surgically inserted to drain the excess CSF from the Ventricles to another body cavity
- Symptoms of acquired hydrocephalus may include altered mental status such as decreased Arousal, Lethargy, confusion, and Frontal Lobe signs; in congenital hydrocephalus cognitive development may be significantly affected including decreased Intelligence and visual-spatial impairments

Hyperacusis. An increased sensitivity to noise that may result from TBI.

Hypersomnolence. Excessive sleeping; can be the result of neurologic trauma, medication side effects, Depression, or other systemic medical disorders; a common initial complaint in persons who have sustained a Mild TBI.

Hypoglossal Nerve. Cranial Nerve XII controls normal tongue movements involved in swallowing and speech; it is actually a pair of nerves that innervates ipsilateral tongue muscles; if one Hypoglossal Nerve is injured, that side of the tongue would be weak, so that when protruded it would deviate toward the weakened or lesioned side.

Hyponatremia. A low sodium (Na^{+}) concentration in the body that may result in thirst, impaired taste sensation, muscle cramps, weakness, Lethargy, confusion, Delirium, Ataxia, Seizures, and even death.

Hypothalamus. A Subcortical Structure that lies below the Thalamus and forms the floor and part of the lateral wall of the third Ventricle; it regulates important physiological drives such as appetite, thirst, sexual arousal, rage, and fear reactions; damage to the Hypothalamus may result in obesity, diminished drive states, altered temperature control, Mood disorders, and explosive disorders; the proximity of the Hypothalamus to other brain structures important for Memory suggests that it may also play some role in that function.

Hypothyroidism. A disturbance of the thyroid that can result in altered cognition (slowed mental thinking, poor Concentration, decreased Memory, sleepiness) and Mood (Depression); replacement therapy often results in total reversal of symptoms.

Hypoxia. Reduced or diminished oxygen supply to the brain; See Anoxia.

Hysteria. A disorder in which there may be neurologic symptoms and dysfunction but without any known physiological cause and presumed to be due to psychological factors.

Illusion. The misperception or misinterpretation of an actual external stimulus (e.g., believing a shadow on the wall is a person walking); illusions differ from Hallucinations in which there is no real or external stimulus.

Impulsivity. Initiating or performing an activity too quickly or without proper planning; a problem of self-regulating behavior that can adversely affect a person's ability to live independently, perform daily activities safely, and work; may also be associated with problems with Attention and distractibility; a common sequela to TBI and Right Hemisphere damage; it may accompany damage to the Frontal Lobes; see Executive Functions.

Treatment of Impulsivity

- Ensure that patient is no longer in Posttraumatic Amnesia, delirious, or in a confusional state as impulse control problems will generally not be amenable to treatment during these times
- Rule out Anxiety problems as Anxiety can increase impulsivity
- Assess and improve patient's Awareness of impulse control problems (e.g., is he or she aware of the impulsivity and its effects on safety?)
- Bring to the patient's attention concrete examples of impulsivity as they occur, how they are related to his or her brain injury, and how they affect daily functioning
- Consider videotaping the patient performing an activity to demonstrate his or her problems in this area
- Treat in a quiet, distraction-free environment
- Model appropriate self-regulation by speaking and moving slowly when dealing with the patient
- Ask the patient to state the task demands (i.e., what he or she is supposed to do) before the maneuver or activity is attempted
- Problem solve with patients what they think will assist them to help them to slow down
- Ask patients how they think their impulsivity will interfere with an activity before they begin it

- Agree with the patient on a specific word such as "Now" or "Go" that will be used by the therapists to signal when to start the activity; stress that the patient is *not* to start an activity until that specific word is said
- Make clear with patients when they are to be listening and when they are to be moving or beginning an activity
- Place a sign in front of patient that reads "Slow Down," "STOP," etc.
- Use visual cues and gestures, such as holding up the hand to indicate "stop," to remind patients to slow down
- Have patients say aloud or to themselves "slow down" or "wait" before beginning an activity
- Have patients pause between each step of an activity by taking a deep breath or saying a word or phrase (such as "easy does it" or "slow down") to themselves or aloud to interrupt the impulsivity
- Give frequent praise and reinforcement to patients when they demonstrate any progress, effort, or insight into their impulsive behaviors
- Give patients concrete examples and praise for any demonstration of improved impulse control
- Use touch to refocus the patient's Attention and to inhibit impulsivity
- Use time estimation activities to help patients more accurately monitor the passage of time as this may improve sustained Attention and slow down rate of thinking
- Use table-top Attention retraining and Cognitive Rehabilitation activities

Inattention. Refers to an inability to attend to a side of the body or an area of space contralateral to the site of the brain lesion; occurs most frequently with nondominant Parietal Lobe damage; see Neglect.

Individualized Educational Program (IEP). An educational plan designed by the public school which outlines the learning needs of the child, including the amount of special education or resource help to be provided, the educational and learning goals, and the frequency of the interventions within the school; it usually is revised yearly; the parents of the child must be in agreement with the IEP in order for it to be instituted; special education help for children with TBI should be included in the IEP.

Infarct. An area of necrosis or dead tissue resulting from an insufficient blood supply.

Information Subtest. A subtest on the Wechsler Adult Intelligence Scale—Revised and on the Wechsler Intelligence Scale for Children—III that assesses general knowledge; in older individuals it can reflect long term or remote Memory; performance is affected by educational level; this subtest tends to be generally resistant to the effects of acquired brain injury unless language skills are damaged.

Initiation. See Abulia.

Insight. See Awareness.

Insomnia. The inability to sleep which may be the result of psychological factors, such as Anxiety, Mania, or Depression, or which may result from organic causes, such as brain injury, Cerebrovascular Accidents, medication effects, or Dementia; insomnia may occur at the beginning, middle, or end of the sleep cycle; see Sleep Disorders.

Intelligence. A multidimensional concept that refers generally to a person's ability to understand complex ideas, adapt effectively to the environment, learn from experience, and engage in various forms of reasoning.

- It comprises several different abilities, some of which are "measured" by intelligence tests, but others such as creativity, practical sense, and social sensitivity are not
- Intelligence is related to higher achievement in school, higher levels of occupational functioning, and more proficient performance on measures of neuropsychological or cognitive functioning such as Memory, Mental Speed, etc. (this relationship, however, is far from perfect)

- Intelligence likely results from both biological and environmental factors
- Intelligence, as measured by Intelligence Tests, generally does not change significantly with mild to moderate brain injury in adults
- Severe brain damage in children can result in significantly lowered intelligence levels
- See Intelligence Tests and IQ.

Neisser, U., Boodoo, G., Bouchard, T. J., et al. (1996). Intelligence: Knowns and unknowns. *American Psychologist, 51,* 77–101.

Intelligence Tests. Psychological tests designed to measure abilities related to the concept of Intelligence; see Intelligence and IQ.

- The most commonly used individual intelligence tests are the Wechsler intelligence scales (Wechsler Adult Intelligence Scale—Revised, Wechsler Intelligence Scale for Children—III, Wechsler Preschool and Primary Scale of Intelligence—Revised) which are composed of verbal and nonverbal subtests yielding a Verbal IQ, a Performance IQ, and a Full Scale IQ
- Other tests provide IQ estimates by measuring more specific functions such as nonverbal abilities only (e.g., Test of Nonverbal Intelligence—2; Raven's Colored or Progressive Matrices) or verbal skills (e.g., Peabody Picture Vocabulary Test—Revised)
- Performance on intelligence tests can be affected by cultural, environmental, and educational factors
- Intelligence tests do *not* measure the effects of acquired brain injury well; there are no real measures of short-term Memory or mental processing speed on intelligence tests, abilities that are frequently disrupted in TBI

Internal Capsule. A crescent shaped collection of White Matter fibers that lie between the Thalamus and the globus pallidus of the Basal Ganglia (see Subcortical Structures).

Internal Carotid Artery. A major artery that supplies blood to the Anterior structures of the brain as it enters the

Circle of Willis and divides into the Anterior Cerebral Artery and the Middle Cerebral Artery (see Cerebral Circulation).

Intracerebral Hemorrhage (ICH). A Hemorrhage or bleed within the brain usually due to hypertension; the ICH may cause focal cognitive and physical deficits depending on the site of the Hemorrhage (unlike Subarachnoid Hemorrhages which tend to result in more diffuse cognitive impairments, particularly with Memory); common sites for ICHs are the Thalamus, Pons, Basal Ganglia, and Cerebellum.

Intracranial Pressure (ICP). The amount of pressure (measured in millimeters of mercury [Hg]) within the cranial vault; increased ICP (>20 mm Hg) occurs frequently in severe TBI due to bleeding within the brain or generalized cerebral swelling (edema) and may cause diffuse brain Ischemia; with high levels of ICP, there may be brain Herniation or a downward or lateral displacement of the brain causing compression of important brain structures, such as the Brain Stem, which can result in death.

IQ. Intelligence Quotient; a derived score from an Intelligence Test that is hypothesized to reflect an objective assessment of an individual's Intelligence

- IQ scores are based on a mean (average) of 100 and a standard deviation of 15
- The average range IQ falls between 90 to 110 which reflects the 25th to the 75th percentiles
- For the Wechsler intelligence scales, less than 70 falls in the mental retardation range
- IQ scores of 80–89 are low average
- IQ scores of 110–119 are high average
- IQ scores above 120 are considered superior
- IQ scores are affected by education and cultural factors
- IQ in adults is not necessarily affected by brain injury
- See also Intelligence, Intelligence Tests, and Test Scores

Ischemia. A lack of blood supply.

Jakob-Creutzfeldt Disease. A rapidly progressive, transmissible disease caused by a poorly understood and complex infectious particle that results in Dementia, myoclonus, Insomnia, and visual complaints; most neurodiagnostic studies are negative; death usually results in 6–12 months.

Judgment of Line Orientation Test. A nonmotor measure of Perceptual Functioning in which the individual is required to match angles of varying degrees to a model; this test is sensitive to Dementia and to Right Hemisphere lesions, particularly Posterior damage.

Benton, A. L., Varney, N. R., & Hamsher, K. (1978). Visuospatial judgment: A clinical test. *Archives of Neurology, 35*, 364–367.

Katz Adjustment Scale: Relative's Form. A scale designed to assess a patient's personal, interpersonal, and social adjustment as seen from a relative's perspective; it consists of several subscales designed to assess a patient's adjustment in such areas as sleep, fears, preoccupations, social performance, household chores, and leisure time.

Katz, M. M., & Lyerly, S. B. (1963). Methods for measuring adjustment and social behavior in the community: I. Rationale, description, discriminative validity and scale development. *Psychological Reports, 13*, 503–535.

Korsakoff's Syndrome. A condition that typically occurs in chronic alcoholics who have a particularly heavy bout of drinking during which time the person eats little food, which results in thiamine (vitamin B) deficiency (thiamine depletion results in cell death and neuronal dysfunction to those brain areas that are most thiamine dependent [specific nuclei in the Thalamus, Mammillary Bodies, Limbic System])

- Both short-term and long-term Memory impairments are the most striking cognitive deficits
- There is long-term Memory impairment for information that occurred most recently prior to the onset of the syndrome (i.e., there is better recall for events that occurred further back in time than for information that occured closer to the onset of the syndrome)
- The short-term Memory deficit (Anterograde Amnesia) can be profound with very little capability for new learning
- Confabulation can occur during the acute stages.

Kluver-Bucy Syndrome. A rare condition caused by bilateral Temporal Lobe damage affecting the Amygdala (usually from trauma or Herpes Simplex Encephalitis) which can result in Apathy, flattened emotional responses, passivity, indiscriminate oral and tactile explorations of the environment, excessive eating, Amnesia, visual Agnosia, and hypersexuality.

Lability. Abrupt and rapid shifts in Affect (e.g., laughing and crying) that can be caused by neurologic insult or injury; see Affect and Pseudobulbar Affect.

Lateralized Signs. Neurologic or cognitive evidence of damage to one hemisphere or the other; it usually presumes the left hemisphere is dominant for language which is true for nearly all right-handers and for the majority of left-handers.

- Left hemisphere signs may include decreased motor or sensory functioning on the right side of the body, language problems (Aphasia, Alexia, Agraphia), and decreased verbal Memory
- Right Hemisphere signs may include decreased motor or sensory functioning on the left side of body, perceptual impairments, left visual Neglect or Inattention, and decreased visual Memory (see Perceptual Functioning)

Learning Disability (LD). A disability or disorder that occurs when Achievement (e.g., reading, math, written expression, spelling) falls significantly below aptitude (e.g., Intelligence) or grade attainment; it is not due to limited Intelligence (persons with LD may have superior Intelligence); the LD may be specific to only one area, such as reading, with all other academic skills intact; it is presumed to be due to an underlying developmental neurologic problem; treatment usually consists of special eduation help in the problematic area; it is important to know if a child with a TBI has a history of LD in order to accurately assess the effects of TBI on cognitive functioning and to make appropriate recommendations to the school; see Dyslexia, School Placement/Considerations, Individualized Educational Plan.

Lethargy. A level of Arousal; not fully alert; the patient tends to drift off to sleep; may lose train of thought due to fatigue or endurance problems; Attention to the examiner and to the environment will also be decreased.

Libido. Sexual desire; can be decreased due to the physiological effects of neurologic insults (e.g., CVA, Traumatic

Brain Injuries, Dementia, Multiple Sclerosis), psychiatric disorders (e.g., Depression, Anxiety), Adjustment problems (e.g., embarrassment about physical condition, dependence on others), general medical conditions such as chronic pain, diabetes, Hypothyroidism, etc., medication side effects (e.g., antidepressants, antihypertensives, pain medications), and advanced age in some but not all cases; neurologic trauma can also increase libido, although this is less common (see Kluver-Bucy Syndrome), or can increase Disinhibition about sexual behavior (e.g., with Frontal Lobe damage); the Limbic System and Hypothalamus appear most critical in the regulation of sexual drive.

Limbic System. A group of Temporal Lobe-related and Subcortical Structures (the components of which are not universally agreed upon by all authors) that are interconnected and play an important role in emotions and Affect, drive states, Memory, olfaction, and Attention; the components of the limbic system are usually thought to include the Amygdala, Hippocampus, Mammillary Bodies, fornix, Anterior nucleus of the Thalamus, and the Cingulate Gyrus; lesions to the Limbic System may result in Amnesia, Abulia, and altered affective and emotional states.

Line Bisection Task. A task used to elicit spatial Inattention or Neglect by asking the patient to find the midpoint of several horizontal lines of varying lengths drawn on a page; the degree to which the patient does not "see" some of the lines or deviates from center in his or her attempt to bisect the line reflects the severity of the Inattention; this task is used more commonly with persons with Right Hemisphere lesions; this task tends to be less sensitive than some other measures, such as Cancellation Tests, in assessing Inattention.

Locked-in Syndrome. A condition in which the patient is mute and essentially quadraplegic but alert, awake, and with intact cognitive functioning.

- Lesions to the Pons or Medulla from infarcts of the Basilar Artery may cause this disorder as well as peripheral nervous system diseases that affect both the Cranial Nerves and the peripheral nerves, such as Guillain-Barré Syndrome or amyotrophic lateral sclerosis
- Because higher cortical structures are intact, cognition is normal
- Careful assessment of the patient's mental status can be accomplished by using the patient's eye blinks or movements to develop a communication system
- This syndrome should not be confused with Coma, Coma Vigil, or a Persistent Vegetative State.

Lumbar Puncture (LP). A neurologic diagnostic test in which a needle is inserted between the lumbar vertebrae into the Subarachnoid space for the purpose of drawing out and examining the Cerebrospinal Fluid; it is particularly helpful in the diagnosis of Meningitis and other infectious illnesses that may affect the central nervous system.

Luria-Nebraska Neuropsychological Battery (LNNB). A standardized neuropsychological assessment battery that was developed in an attempt to incorporate the neuropsychological theory of brain organization and function of Alexandr Luria, a prominent Russian neuropsychologist; the LNNB is divided into 11 subscales; some critics have argued against its diagnostic usefulness.

Golden, C. J., Purish, A. D., & Hammeke, T. A. (1985). *Luria-Nebraska Neuropsychological Battery: Forms I and II.* Los Angeles: Western Psychological Services.

Lyme Disease. A tick-borne, multisystem spirochetal illness that may cause neurologic symptoms including Memory impairment, difficulty with Concentration, Sleep disturbance, irritability, fatigue, and emotional Lability; the Memory impairment appears to reflect problems more with retrieval than storage; antibiotic treatment may eliminate the symptoms although some patients continue to demonstrate cognitive and other problems even with appropriate intervention.

Magnetic Resonance Imaging (MRI). A neuroimaging procedure in which magnetic fields are used to produce computer generated images of body structures of high resolution; it is superior to CT scans in its clarity and because it produces images free of interference from the skull, however, the patient must be capable of lying still for 30–45 minutes and must be free of any metallic devices such as surgical clips, life support, etc.; MRIs are not used for emergency assessment.

Malingering. The intentional production or exaggeration of physical or psychological symptoms motivated by external incentives such as obtaining financial compensation in a lawsuit or avoiding unpleasant circumstances such as prison; malingering should be suspected if patients misrepresent their history, exhibit deficits that far exceed the parameters of their injury, develop symptoms well beyond the time that problems usually develop from similar injuries in other people, or if they are reluctant to provide records or information from previous health care providers; face-to-face interviews are often ineffective in detecting malingering; the exaggeration of cognitive deficits must be assessed by measures designed specifically to evaluate these types of problems (e.g., forced choice procedures, symptom validity testing).

Guilmette, T. J., & Bishop, D. S. (1994). Malingering. In E. Feldmann (Ed.), *Current diagnosis in neurology* (pp. 304–307). St. Louis, MO: Mosby-Year Book, Inc.

Mammillary Bodies. Two adjacent pea-sized white masses that make up the posterior portion of the Hypothalamus and that, along with the Hippocampus and the Thalamus, are involved with Memory; they are part of the Limbic System (see Subcortical Structures).

Mania. The presence of elevated, expansive, or irritable Mood (e.g., inflated self-esteem, decreased need for sleep, increased motor activity, increased verbal activity, racing thoughts); when accompanied by periods of Depression, it is referred to as Manic-Depressive or Bipolar Disorder; the incidence of mania following TBI is generally unknown but has been reprted in one study in up to 9% of persons postinjury, particularly with those with Anterior Temporal Lobe lesions; mania may also occur in persons with Multiple Sclerosis, Huntington's Disease, and other neurologic disorders.

Jorge, R. E., Robinson, R. G., Starkstein, S. E., Arndt, S. V., Forrester, A. W., & Geisler, F. R. (1993). Secondary mania following traumatic brain injury. *American Journal of Psychiatry, 150,* 916–921.

Mass Effect. A condition in which brain structures are "pushed" or displaced due to swelling or an intracerebral mass such as a Hemorrhage or Tumor; this can occur because brain tissue is relatively soft and because there is no room for the brain to expand due to the confines of the skull.

Mazes. Maze tracing tests are designed to assess planning and organization, abilities that can be adversely affected by TBI due to Impulsivity and poor organizational skills; in children, the most commonly used maze test is the Mazes subtest of the Wechsler Intelligence Scale for Children—III; the Porteus Maze Test is another maze tracing test used with both children and adults.

Medulla. The lowest part of the Brain Stem which is important for the regulation of respiration, blood pressure, and heart rate; it is also known as the bulb; see Bulbar Nerves.

Medulloblastoma. The most common Posterior fossa Tumor found in children; it is usually situated in the Cerebellum and infiltrates the fourth Ventricle resulting in increased Intracranial Pressure; surgical removal and radiation therapy significantly improve survival rates; cognitive deficits and some behavioral changes can occur due to the effects of surgery and radiation.

Memory. The ability to absorb (i.e., learn), retain, and recall information derived from our experiences.

- Memory is a highly complex and not well understood cognitive process

- The ability to learn and retain new information results from an interaction of many brain and cognitive systems, particularly a person's Arousal, Attention, sensory functioning (e.g., vision, hearing), Motivation, and reasoning skills
- Memory is not likely a unitary system, but rather, can be divided into several subsystems
- Brain structures that appear most important for new learning include the Hippocampus, Thalamus, Frontal Lobes, Mammillary Bodies, and other components of the Limbic System (see Subcortical Structures)
- Frontal Lobe damage specifically tends to produce deficits with retrieval (and not storage) of new information, impaired recall of temporal order (i.e., recalling which information was learned first, second, etc.), under which circumstances new material was presented, and defective Awareness and insight about memory problems
- Learning and memory can be affected by almost any neurologic disorder that affects brain functioning although the most significant Amnesias (i.e., memory loss) tend to result from Anoxia, Korsakoff's Syndrome, Alzheimer's Disease and other Dementias, Herpes Simplex Encephalitis, Subarachnoid Hemorrhages, and Traumatic Brain Injury
- In TBI, memory impairment is more common in patients with longer periods of Coma and Posttraumatic Amnesia, lower admitting Glasgow Coma Scale scores, and Anoxia at the time of trauma
- Patients with memory disorders have difficulty generalizing information learned in one context to another
- Figure 6 outlines a tentative memory taxonomy in which memory is generally divided along two dimensions: *declarative* (information that can be "declared" or brought to mind as an idea, image, word, or fact) and *Procedural* (memory that is retained as a learned skill, motor response, or cognitive operation); episodic memory refers to memory for the past event's of one's life (Autobio-

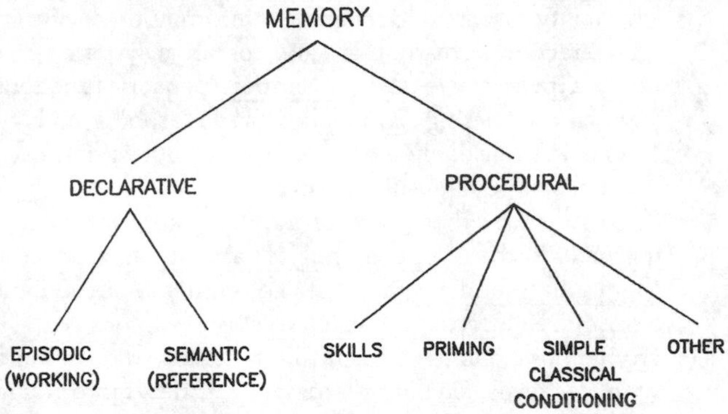

Figure 6. A tentative memory taxonomy (Reprinted with permission from *Memory and Brain* by L. R. Squire, 1987, p. 170. Copyright 1987 by Oxford University Press, Inc.)

graphical Memory) and semantic memory refers to knowledge and facts about the world

- Declarative memory is affected by Amnesia but Procedural Learning is not; thus patients can learn skills and procedures through repetitve practice even if a significant Amnesia is present

Clinical Aspects of Memory

- ***Immediate Memory:*** the temporary holding or storage of information necessary for such complex cognitive tasks as language comprehension, learning, and reasoning
  - May also be known as "working memory" although it is more dependent on Attention than memory
  - It is a necessary first step in the stages of short-term memory
  - Immediate memory lasts generally from about 30 seconds to perhaps a few minutes, long enough to decide what to do with the information

- Its capacity is generally believed to be five to nine pieces of information at a time
- It is most impaired in patients with severe attentional disorders such as Delirium
- Patients with Amnesia usually have intact immediate memory spans
- Testing of immediate memory can be done with digit spans, recall of sentences, and recall of the first trial of a word list

- ***Short-term Memory (STM):*** a general term for the retention of information over a short time or after brief distraction
  - May also be known as recent memory, delayed memory, delayed recall, or anterograde memory
  - Information enters short-term memory from the immediate memory span
  - The duration of STM may be hours to weeks
  - It is facilitated by rehearsal and practice
  - Information that is more emotionally charged or important is more easily stored in short-term memory
  - Short-term memory is the type of memory that is most impaired in Amnesia (a severe short-term memory deficit is also known as Anterograde Amnesia) and is contingent upon such brain structures as the Hippocampus, Thalamus, Frontal Lobes, Mammillary Bodies, and the Limbic System
  - Short-term memory is the type of memory most vulnerable to neurologic injury and is most affected by TBI, Anoxia, Korsakoff's Syndrome, Herpes Simplex Encephalitis, Alzheimer's Disease and other Dementias, and Subarachnoid Hemorrhage
  - STM can be affected by age (see Age Effects)
  - During Posttraumatic Amnesia, STM is the dimension of memory most affected
  - Information in STM may be transferred or consolidated to long-term memory (if STM is deficient, then information will not be transferred or stored in long-term memory)

  - The assessment of STM can be accomplished with many different types of memory measures, including the Memory Assessment Scales, Wechsler Memory Scale—Revised, California or Rey Auditory Verbal Learning Tests, Benton Visual Retention Test, and many others
  - In children, STM can be assessed with the Wide Range Assessment of Memory and Learning (WRAML), Test of Memory and Learning (TOML), and the California or Rey Auditory Verbal Learning Tests
- ***Longterm Memory (LTM):*** information that is stored and retained over a longer time frame such as months, years, or a lifetime
  - LTM may also be known as remote memory or distant memory and also includes Autobiographical Memory (i.e., information about oneself and one's personal history)
  - In persons with memory disorders following brain injury, recent memory usually refers to information learned or presented after the onset of the disorder and remote memory usually refers to information acquired before the disorder (recent memory is more often impaired than remote memory)
  - STM must be relatively intact for new information to be stored in or transferred to LTM (thus, if STM is impaired, "new" long-term memories cannot be created either)
  - Information in LTM is *least* resistant to deterioration following neurologic insult or injury; it is usually the most preserved type of memory in persons with severe memory impairment (e.g., Alzheimer's Disease, Anoxia)
  - If LTM is impaired, then STM is also very likely to be deficient
  - There is not necessarily a clear distinction or time frame for when STM ends and LTM begins
  - There is much less known about the underlying neuroanatomy necessary for LTM than for STM although the Thalamus appears to play some role in this function

- Assessing LTM is usually done less formally than with STM; questions about the person's past can be asked, recall of cultural events that happened before the onset of the neurologic disorder can be ascertained (e.g., past presidents, important historical events that occurred during the person's lifetime), and assessment of older abilities and skills can be conducted

- ***Visual versus Verbal Memory:*** Visual memory is memory for information that is not language based and is processed by the brain with little or no language component (e.g., designs, images), whereas verbal memory is memory for information that is language dependent, regardless of whether it is spoken or written
  - Information is rarely only verbal or visual, rather, it may be processed in both modalities
  - Many visual memory tasks (e.g., the ability to memorize drawings or designs) can be aided by language and by the brain interpreting the visual stimulus verbally (i.e., translating what it "sees" into words)
  - In some cases, one type of memory may be more deficient than the other due to injury and the other type of memory may be a relative strength
  - Although the brain works as a whole unit in processing information, in most persons the left hemisphere is dominant for verbal memory and the Right Hemisphere is dominant for visual memory; thus a left hemisphere injury may result in greater verbal then visual memory impairment and a Right Hemisphere injury may result in greater visual than verbal memory impairment

- ***Rate of Learning:*** Refers to how quickly a person can absorb new information
  - Highly dependent on Attention, Concentration, and Mental Speed
  - Can be affected by Depression and Anxiety
  - Patients with memory disorders may be able to learn and absorb new information but at reduced rates and efficiency

- Persons with TBI frequently learn new information more slowly and inefficiently than persons without TBI
- If rate of learning is impaired, then repetition and additional time to absorb the new information can be helpful
- A patient must have learned or absorbed the new information initially in order to determine if he or she retained or stored it over time

- ***Recall/Retrieval Versus Recognition/Storage:*** Recall/retrieval of information refers to a person's ability to spontaneously or freely recall information upon demand whereas recognition/storage refers to a person's ability to identify the information previously learned when given cues or multiple choices, which reflects how well the material was stored by the brain
  - Recall is assessed by asking patients to recall information they had previously learned, either recently to evaluate short-term memory or for events that happened long ago to assess long-term memory
  - If patients do not spontaneously recall or retrieve information well it does not necessarily mean that it has been forgotten; information can be stored but may not be immediately accessible for recall
  - Assessing how well information is stored or retained requires that recognition memory be evaluated; give patients cues or multiple choices to determine if they can identify information they had known in the past or been exposed to recently; if recognition improves recall, then the information has been stored, if it does not help, then the information is truly forgotten
  - Retrieval or recall deficits are relatively common sequelae to many neurologic insults, particularly with Frontal Lobe injuries, and are frequently observed as an Aging Effect
  - Retrieval or recall deficits are less debilitating than storage impairments and respond more favorably to memory retraining and other Cognitive Rehabilitation strategies

- Recognition or storage deficits are the most functionally debilitating type of memory impairment and are more likely to occur with Anoxia, Korsakoff's Syndrome, Alzheimer's Disease, Herpes Simplex Encephalitis, in the acute stages of Subarachnoid Hemorrhages, and during acute recovery from TBI or Posttramatic Amnesia
- Recognition or storage deficits are usually accompanied by very poor Awareness or insight about the memory disorder and require the use of compensatory memory aids/reminders such as lists, notes, Memory Log, etc.

General Treatment Suggestions for Memory Disorders

- Begin with a thorough and comprehensive assessment of the patient's cognitive functions, particularly Attention and Concentration, and memory capacities (e.g., rate of learning, recall, retention and storage, visual and verbal)
- Patients will not respond well to any formal memory retraining if they are Agitated, highly inattentive (e.g., in a Delirium), or completely unmotivated
- Rule out Aphasia or severe perceptual disorders that may interfere with new learning for verbal or visual information, respectively
- Determine patients' Awareness of their memory functioning (known as metamemory) and intervene as necessary to improve insight (also see Cognitive Rehabilitation entry); without Awareness, patients will be more difficult to engage in treatment and to use rehabilitation strategies
- Identify the strengths and weaknesses of the patient's memory/cognitive functioning and determine which specific aspects of the patient's memory are impaired and need to be addressed
- Use more intact areas of cognitive functions and memory to supplement weaker memory skills
- Review and reinforce with patients their autobiographical and long-term memory (i.e., date of birth, age, home address, names/ages of children, age of spouse, length of

marriage, previous jobs, etc.) and Orientation information before any formal memory rehabilitation for current or recent events is undertaken (long-term memory should be more accessible and more easily cued than any other type of memory or information)

- Attention is crucial for learning new information; ensure that patients are being attentive before new information is given to them
- Teach patients to anticipate when and in what way their memory problems may interfere with new learning and what they must do for themselves to learn and retain information better
- Prompt patients verbally and nonverbally before new information or techniques are going to be given to them (e.g. use statements such as, "This is important so I want you to try to remember how we're doing this.")
- Be explicit about what patients are expected to remember or to try to memorize
- Speak slowly to patients and give information in small units or chunks
- Have the patients repeat instructions or information that you want them to remember
- Use words, vocabulary, and concepts that patients are familiar with and can understand
- Allow patients time to process and internally rehearse new information
- Determine what information is most critical for the patients to learn and then focus most on that information (this may consist of only two or three concepts such as always using the walker or reaching back for the chair before sitting down); consistency and brevity are crucial for new learning in patients with memory disorders
- All staff must teach patients in the same way, using the same words, the same steps to each task, and the same instructions; the patient must practice each new technique in the same way each time in order to optimize learning

- For patients who are not overly concrete, explain the rationale for what you want the patient to remember and why; people often learn better if they understand the context of information presented to them and how it fits into their overall treatment plan
- Patients with severe memory disorders can learn if they practice, practice, practice; but the practice and instructions must be the same each time
- When trying to learn new techniques, practice is usually more effective if it occurs over shorter but more frequent sessions than for longer but fewer sessions (i.e., three 20-minute therapy sessions conducted over the course of the day will usually be more effective for new learning than one 60-minute session)
- Include patients in developing memory strategies; ask them what strategy or technique that they think they can use to remember new information
- At the beginning of a new treatment session review with the patient what was practiced or taught at the previous session
- Patients with memory disorders have limited capacity (i.e., they can learn only limited amounts of information at a time) which requires that new learning be focused only on the most important information and techniques
- Prior to beginning a task, review with patients the most important information that they are to remember when performing the activity
- Patients with Amnesia or impaired memory storage have intact Procedural Learning (i.e., skill learning) which means that they are able to learn new techniques such as transfers, ADL skills, ambulation with assistive devices, etc. even though they have no conscious memory of the techniques and cannot explain how to perform the activity if asked; however, in order to learn new skills these patients must practice the activity in the same way over and over again; these patients will learn only by doing and

not by talking about the activity or having it explained frequently to them

- Memory retraining through restorative techniques (e.g., attempts at improving memory through the repetition or drilling of memory tasks such as asking patients to remember lists of words/numbers, stories, etc.) seems to have limited value in improving memory for functional activities; see approaches to Cognitive Rehabilitation
- The most successful interventions for memory impairments, particularly for severe deficits, are generally compensation techniques

Treatment Techniques for Memory Disorders

- Patients with higher level or subtle impairments (e.g., problems with retrieval but not storage) may benefit from using memory strategies or mnemonic techniques; these techniques, however, require effort, practice, and Motivation to use effectively; many of these memory strategies or techniques are described in self-help memory books available at local book stores
  - Visual imagery can be used as a mnemonic strategy by asking patients to visualize scenes which include the information they are to remember (usually the more bizarre or comical the scene, the more easily it will be remembered); a loci method has also been used wherein the person is asked to visualize a home or building and then to imagine that each item that is to be remembered is placed in a different room (when the person wants to recall the item, he or she can do so by mentally moving from room to room to remember the items)
  - Associations can be made between the new information to be remembered and other information that the person already has in storage
  - Rearrange information in a way that will make it easier to remember by using abbreviations, a play on words, etc. (e.g., using the word HOMES to remember the Great Lakes of Huron, Ontario, Michigan, Erie, Superior)

- Enlist patients' participation by asking them to create words or cues that can remind them of longer or more detailed information (e.g., the steps of a transfer or other acitivty can be consolidated into a few words or phrases which can then remind the patient of what he or she is to do next)
- Abbreviate instructions to only one word or a simple phrase so that the word or phrase can act as a cue to remind the patient of a longer command or instruction (e.g., the phrase "reach back" can be reviewed frequently with the patient as a reminder to reach back for the arm of the chair during a transfer for the patient who has trouble remembering to reach back to the chair before sitting down)
- External aids or reminders (memory orthotics) can be very important memory compensation techniques, particularly for patients with severe memory storage deficits; as patients improve the demands on their memory can be increased and the cues to remember can be diminished
  - Write down the steps of an activity to be performed and ask the patient to follow the list during the task; the patient can also review the list when not in therapy
  - Use brief words or phrases (or pictures if language is a weakness) on index cards to guide the patient through an activity; ask the patient to put the cards in their correct order before the activity is begun
  - Use wristwatches with timers to remind patients of important information; computer and electronic devices can also be used although their cost can be prohibitive and patients must feel comfortable with them to use them effectively; generally, the more complicated the device, the less likely patients will use them
  - Use written daily schedules, appointment calendars, pocket notebooks, and <u>Memory Log</u> books to remind them of important information
  - All strategies must be "user-friendly" for the patient to use them when needed and to generalize to situations

outside of treatment; discuss frequently with patients how the memory systems can be refined to meet their needs

Memory Assessment Scales (MAS). A standardized Memory battery for adults that assesses both visual and verbal information in normal and clinical populations.

Williams, J. M. (1991). *Memory Assessment Scales Manual*. Odessa, FL: Psychological Assessment Resources, Inc.

Memory Log. An external, compensatory Memory aid in which patients write down information to be remembered such as their daily schedule, medications, appointments, etc. due to impaired Memory; Memory logs should not be used if the patient is aphasic and unable to read, has impaired visual acuity, is illiterate, has severe perceptual deficits such as Neglect, or exhibits impaired Arousal, severe confusion, or Delirium.

Suggestions for Implementing a Memory Log Book

- Identify the goals and objectives for implementing a Memory log book; what is its purpose?
- Determine what information and how much detail should be contained in the log book
- The greater the level of confusion and impaired Orientation, the less information and details the log book should contain; ascertain how much information and stimulation the patient can tolerate
- Patients with subtler and higher level deficits can often tolerate and require more detail in their log books
- Orienting information may contain very basic details such as the month, year, place, and reason for hospitalization; autobiographical information such as age, date of birth, home address, names/ages of spouses and children will be important to include if the patient is confused about these facts
- For more impaired patients, cover the log book in brightly colored paper or cloth to make it stand out from the other surroundings in their environment

- Help the patient to identify a special place where the log book will be kept when it is not being used
- Have the patient take the log book with him or her to all appointments and therapies
- Use a format and style for the log book that the patient feels comfortable with to increase the likelihood that he or she will use it
- Pictures of treating therapists, the patient's home, family members, etc. can be placed in the log book to facilitate recall of this type of information
- Identify a specific therapist who will be responsible for creating and modifying the log book as necessary
- Educate the family about the rationale and purpose for the log book and enlist their help in reinforcing the proper use of it
- The log book may contain several sections such as calendars/appointments, things to do, medication schedules, maps, etc.
- The patient will need to practice using the log book like any other orthotic device
- Encourage patients to use only one memory aid and to have that with them at all times (due to their Anxiety, patients tend to create mutiple systems such as having a calendar at home, lists of information everywhere, slips of paper in their pockets, etc., which usually results in greater confusion)
- Patients must learn to write down appropriate information in their log and to look at it (without these two fundamental steps [writing and reviewing], the log book will not be effective)
- Help patients develop a schedule for looking at their log book even if they think there is nothing specific they need to remember at that time (using a wristwatch with an alarm can be used as a reminder or teaching them to look at it at specific times of day, e.g., when they wake up, at all the even numbered hours, at mealtime, at bedtime)

Meninges. The three protective membranes that enclose the brain and spinal cord; they include (from outermost to innermost layers) the Dura Mater, the Arachnoid, and the Pia Mater.

Meningioma. A Tumor that arises from the Meninges; they tend to grow slowly and occur almost exclusively in adults; they produce symptoms by compressing on the brain structures underneath them but do not infiltrate other brain tissue; most can be totally removed by surgery.

Meningitis. An infection of the Cerebrospinal Fluid that results in inflammation of the Meninges; may be bacterial, which can be life-threatening, or viral, which is usually more benign; meningitis can result in residual and chronic cognitive deficits in some cases.

Mental Retardation. A classification of mental functioning in which a person's measured Intelligence falls below 70 and is accompanied by significant limitations in adaptive functioning in at least two of the following skill areas: communication, self-care, home living, social/interpersonal skills, use of community resources, self-direction, functional academic skills, work, leisure, health, and safety (DSM-IV criteria); the onset must occur before age 18; most cases of mental retardation are congenital; persons with a normal development who sustain a significant loss of IQ due to TBI, Dementia, or other acquired neurological disorder are not described as mentally retarded.

Mental Speed. The speed and efficiency with which a person is able to process and mentally manipulate information; it is one of the most sensitive areas of cognitive functioning to brain injury and is often impaired following TBI; mental speed can be assessed informally by determining how quickly a person responds to questions and task demands; formal evaluation of mental speed can be accomplished through the Trail Making Test, the Paced Auditory

Serial Addition Test, and other timed measures of cognitive efficiency; it can also be decreased due to Depression; see also Attention and Concentration.

Midbrain. The highest or most forward portion of the Brain Stem; it contains the major portion of the Reticular Activating System; it plays a role in basic facial responses such as crying, laughing, and sucking and has been associated with some movement disorders and tremor; impaired Memory retrieval has been associated with damage to the connecting fibers between the midbrain and other brain structures associated with Memory.

Middle Cerebral Artery (MCA). One of the main sources of blood supply to the cerebral Cortex, the MCA arises from the Circle of Willis and travels along the lateral or outside surface of the brain supplying blood to a large portion of the Temporal Lobes and to portions of the Frontal, Parietal, and Occipital Lobes; it is the most common site of Cerebrovascular Accidents within the brain; lesions to the MCA can cause significant cognitive impairment including Aphasia on the left side and deficits with Perceptual Functioning on the right side; see also Cerebral Circulation.

Midline Shift. A shifting or pushing of the longitudinal fissure (the large groove or sulcus that separates the two cerebral hemispheres) and midline brain structures due to a space occupying lesion (e.g., Tumor, Subdural Hematoma); see also Mass Effect and Herniation.

Mild Traumatic Brain Injury (MTBI). One of the three classifications of severity of Traumatic Brain Injury (the other two being moderate and severe).

- According to the American Congress of Rehabilitation, a patient with MTBI has had a traumatically induced physiological disruption of brain function, as manifested by at least one of the following:
  1. any period of loss of consciousness;

2. any loss of Memory for events immediately before or after the accident;
3. any alteration in mental state at the time of the accident (e.g., feeling dazed, disoriented, or confused); and
4. focal neurological deficit(s) that may or may not be transient; but where the severity of the injury does not exceed the following:
   a. loss of consciousness of approximately 30 minutes or less
   b. after 30 minutes, an initial Glasgow Coma Scale of 13–15; and
   c. Posttraumatic Amnesia not greater than 24 hours

- The most common symptoms generally fall into one of the following categories:
  - *Physical:* headache, dizziness, nausea, sleep problems, fatigue, Photophobia
  - *Cognitive:* decreased Attention, Concentration, Mental Speed, short-term Memory
  - *Emotional:* irritability, emotional Lability, Depression, Anxiety
- The majority of persons who sustain MTBI will recovery spontaneously and without any residual problems within about 1 to 3 months, although some patients may require a somewhat longer time frame
- A small subset of persons with MTBI will be left with permanent disability although the reasons for this are a cause of controversy within the field; it is unclear whether permanent disability is the result of organic or psychological factors (or a complex interaction of the two); Motivation and litigation issues have also been raised as affecting presentation of symptoms
- Because MTBI patients who report long-term sequelae to their injuries have more problems with pain, sleep, and Depression/Anxiety than persons with more severe TBI, the role of these issues in cognitive functioning also needs to be considered

- There is likely a cumulative effect to sustaining multiple brain injuries (i.e., patients may exhibit more or longer lasting problems if they have sustained prior brain injuries)
- Outcome may be worse for patients involved in high speed motor vehicle accidents and for those with histories of substance abuse, psychiatric disorders, limited premorbid functioning, or if they are older
- Neuroimaging, such as CT scans and Magnetic Resonance Imaging, and standard neurologic exams are often negative in MTBI

Treatment Suggestions for Mild Traumatic Brain Injury

- Educate patients about MTBI symptoms; normalize their experience (e.g., "Headaches are very common with this type of injury and are a normal part of the recovery process")
- Provide reassurance and support
- Predict a good recovery with time (i.e., the majority of people recover fully in about 1–3 months)
- Help patients to manage stress in their lives and to prioritize their daily activities
- Give patients permission to temporarily avoid stressful and cognitively demanding tasks but encourage them to remain as intellectually active as they feel able to
- Avoid alcohol during the recovery process
- Encourage patients to get plenty of rest
- Help patients compensate for the temporary disruption of their cognitive functions by using external Memory aids, such as lists and Memory Logs, and by structuring their environment to decrease distraction and to limit external stimuli
- Monitor Mood and Anxiety; refer for treatment if necessary
- Refer patient for treatment of pain and sleep problems if necessary
- Educate family members about the usual sequelae of MTBI and how they can assist the patient during the recovery process

- Suggest that patients not make any significant life decisions for the first few months after their injury

Gualtieri, T. C. (1995). The problem of mild brain injury. *Neuropsychiatry, Neuropsychology, and Behavioral Neurology, 8,* 127–136.

Kay, T. (1993). Neuropsychological treatment of mild traumatic brain injury. *Journal of Head Trauma Rehabilitation, 8,* 74–85.

Leininger, B. E., Gramling, S. E., Farrell, A. D., Kreutzer, J. S., & Peck, E. A. (1990). Neuropsychological deficits in symptomatic minor head injury patients after concussion and mild concussion. *Journal of Neurology, Neurosurgery, and Psychiatry, 53,* 293–296.

Mild Traumatic Brain Injury Committee of the Head Injury Interdisciplinary Special Interest Group of the American College of Rehabilitation Medicine. (1993). Definition of mild traumatic brain injury. *Journal of Head Injury Rehabilitation, 8,* 86–87.

Youngjohn, J. R., Burrows, L., & Erdal, K. (1995). Brain damage or compensation neurosis? The controversial post-concussion syndrome. *The Clinical Neuropsychologist, 9,* 112–123.

Mini-Mental State Examination (MMS). A popular mental status screening measure that provides a very brief assessment of Orientation, Attention, Memory, and Constructional Ability; it is based on a 0–30 scoring system; it was originally designed to assess Dementia in psychiatric populations; research suggests that it may be insensitive to specific brain lesions, Amnesia, and mild cognitive deficits; a score less than 24 has been associated with Dementia; it should not be used alone when a comprehensive cognitive assessment is necessary for diagnostic or treatment purposes.

Folstein, M. F., Folstein, S. E., & McHugh, P. R. (1975). 'Mini-Mental State': A practical method for grading cognitive state of patients for the clinicians. *Journal of Psychiatric Research, 12,* 189–198.

Minnesota Multiphasic Personality Inventory (MMPI). The best known and most researched objective measure of Personality and emotional functioning used in psychological testing; it is sensitive to many emotional disorders that may be exacerbated by result from neurologic illness or disease; it has also been shown to be sensitive in Malingering detection.

Modified Mini-Mental State Examination (3MS). A brief screening measure of mental or cognitive functioning; it is an expanded version of the Mini-Mental State Examination (MMS) which taps a broader range of cognitive abilities including verbal fluency, delayed Memory with recognition, remote personal information, and abstraction; the score range is 0–100; the 3MS has been found to provide additional cognitive information and better prediction of functional outcome than the MMS in a geriatric stroke population.

Grace, J., Nadler, J. D., White, D. A., Guilmette, T. J., Giuliano, A. J., Monsch, A. U., & Snow, M. G. (1995). Folstein vs Modified Mini-Mental State Examination in geriatric stroke. *Archives of Neurology, 52,* 477–484.

Teng, E. L., & Chui, H. C. (1987). The Modified Mini-Mental State (3MS) Examination. *Journal of Clinical Psychiatry, 48,* 314–318.

Mood. A pervasive and sustained emotional state such as Depression, Anxiety, irritability, etc.; mood may be altered directly by neurologic or brain insults or in reaction/adjustment to a person's disability; mood disorders must be carefully monitored during rehabilitation and treated, if necessary, as they can adversely affect participation in rehabilitation, cognitive abilities, social interaction, Family Functioning, frustration tolerance, etc.; mood may be affected by the patient's insight or Awareness into his or her deficits (e.g., less insight usually results in fewer mood problems) and by lesions to the Limbic System or other brain structures; see also Affect and Adjustment.

Examples of Mood

- *Dysphoric mood:* Unpleasant mood such as sadness, irritability, etc.
- *Elevated mood:* An exaggerated feeling of well-being, euphoria, or elation
- *Euthymic mood:* Mood in the "normal" range, which implies an absence of Depression or elevated mood
- *Expansive mood:* Lack of restraint in expressing one's feelings, frequently with an overvaluation of one's significance or importance; see Mania

- *Irritable mood:* Easily annoyed or provoked to anger

American Psychiatric Association. (1994). *Diagnostic and statistical manual of mental disorders* (4th ed.). Washington, DC: Author.

Motivation. A complex interaction of psychological and physiological processes that result in an individual's desire, drive, or motive to perform a certain acitivity, pursue a plan of action, participate in treatment, etc.

- Motivation in rehabilitation can be affected by a host of factors including brain trauma (particularly with damage to the Frontal Lobes and some Subcortical Structures), premorbid Personality, emotional functioning and Mood, environmental and social issues, medical status, medication side effects, Awareness of deficits and need for treatment, hope for recovery, expectations for treatment, and perceived benefit of rehabilitation
- Increasing motivation may be a specific goal of rehabilitation treatment (see Abulia)
- It must be considered in all rehabilitation plans as patients' motivation for treatment will affect their participation with therapists, their willingness to use compensatory strategies, to use orthotic or assistive devices, etc.

Suggestions for Increasing Motivation in Rehabilitation

- Assess reasons for the patient's lack of motivation
  - Is there a premorbid history of poor compliance with following medical advice or in taking instructions from others?
  - Is there evidence of injury to specific brain structures that may affect drive?
  - Does the patient have a history of needing to be in control or in charge?
  - Is there a history of passive-aggressive traits (i.e., a tendency to express anger and resentment through passive behavior), overdependence on others, or an external locus of control (i.e., the belief that a person cannot control his or her own future and that "fate" completely determines what happens to us)?

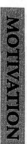

- Is the patient depressed or anxious?
- Are there any Personality conflicts between the patient and treating staff?
- Does the patient have confidence in those treating him or her?
- Does the patient feel comfortable in the physical environment of the rehabilitation setting?
- Is the patient physically ill?
- Is there a pain problem interfering with treatment?
- Is the patient bothered by excessive fatigue or poor endurance?
- Are there medications that are interfering with the patient's compliance or drive?
- Is the patient aware of his or her deficits and how they affect his or her functioning?
- Does the patient understand the rationale for and agree with the treatment plan?
- Does the patient believe that he or she will get better and that treatment will improve his or her ability to function and his or her quality of life?
- Is the patient hopeful and optimistic about the future?
- Are the patient's expectations for treatment consistent with the treatment itself?
- Is the patient expecting a "miracle cure"?
- Are the patient's expectations for improvement accurate (i.e., does he or she believe that improvement is gradual or that it will happen all-at-once)?
- Does the patient believe that he or she is getting better?
- Are the patient's goals consistent with the goals of the rehabilitation team?
- Is the patient constantly comparing him- or herself with how he or she used to be before the injury rather than the progress he or she has made since the injury?
- Is the patient's family in agreement with the goals and treatment plan?
- Is the family encouraging of the patient?

- See Abulia entry for treatment of severe organic amotivational disorders
- Engage patient in the treatment planning process; ensure that the treatment goals are compatible with the patient's desires
- Correct any erroneous expectations about recovery or how progress occurs (patients may believe that recovery stops at a specific time or that it happens suddenly, e.g., when they wake up some morning)
- Continue to give patients hope about future recovery
- Give patients as much information as they can understand about their disorder, rationale for treatment, and expectations for improvement
- Increase patients' Awareness of their deficits, their effects on daily functioning and quality of life, and how treatment will facilitate recovery and make their life better (see Awareness entry); this issue can be critical in enhancing a patient's willingness to engage in treatment
- Treat Depression and Anxiety; patients may require a referral to a mental health professional, including a psychiatrist for medication
- Give patients choices in their treatment (e. g., "Which activity would you like to do first?" or "Would you like to do this now or later?")
- Give patients as much control over their treatment as possible and include them in making decisions about therapeutic activities
- Have patients write their long- and short-term goals on a sheet of paper, tape them on a wall where they will see them often, and have them ask themselves the questions, "What did I do today (or what am I going to do today) to reach my goals?" and "What could I have done differently (or what am I going to do differently) to reach my goals?"
- Let the therapist who has the best relationship with the patient and whom the patient trusts most discuss motivation and compliance issues with the patient

- Enlist the family in encouraging the patient and in helping the patient understand the need for treatment (remember that just because you may be the "expert," there is no intrinsic reason why the patient should trust someone he or she doesn't know)
- Build patients' trust by listening to them and trying to understand their point of view
- Do not "order" a patient to perform an activity as this will usually serve to increase resistance
- Respond to the patient's psychological needs (e.g., for control or dependence) with the realization that there will likely need to be compromise on both the part of the patient and the staff to increase compliance
- With a resistant patient, ask yourself, "Why should the patient comply . . . what's in it for him or her?"; what will motivate the patient and what will the patient work for? (see Behavior Management entry)
- Try Behavior Contracts to increase compliance and motivation
- Attend to the medical needs of the patient; investigate complaints of fatigue, pain, poor sleep, physical discomfort, etc.

Motor Strip. Controls voluntary movements of skeletal muscles on the opposite side of the body; it is located in the most Posterior portion of the Frontal Lobes (the first Gyrus Anterior to the Central Sulcus); it is also known as the primary motor cortex; see Cerebrum.

Multi-infarct Dementia. A global term for a Dementia caused by multiple Infarcts (Cerebrovascular Accidents) in the brain; onset of neurologic symptoms is usually acute with a period of remission or stable symptoms followed again by more neurologic deficits (this is referred to as a "step-wise" deterioration due to the effect of each successive stroke); cognitive impairments may vary with a scattering of deficits interspersed with relatively preserved functioning in some areas; eventually, with more strokes, greater cognitive impairments become apparent; hypertension and diabetes are common risk factors; for treatment considerations refer to Dementia entry.

Multiple Sclerosis (MS). One of the most common disabling neurologic disorders in adults in which the myelin sheaths (the White Matter covering of the Axons which facilitates transmission of nerve impulses) become episodically inflamed and eventually stripped away from the neuron; onset is usually between ages 15 and 50; there is no known cause or cure.

- The most common physical MS symptoms include weakness, sensory disturbances, Ataxia, ocular impairments, bladder and sexual dysfunction, and generalized physical and mental exhaustion
- The course of the disorder is marked by the unpredictable acute exacerbation of symptoms followed by relatively stable periods of fewer or less intense symptoms
- MS progresses at different rates for different people
- Depression is understandably the most common emotional response although some patients may also develop a euphoric state in which their Mood is elevated (sometimes referred to as MS euphoria) and they have limited insight or Awareness into their own deficits or needs
- The cognitive disturbances associated with MS are dependent upon the randomness of where and to what extent the demyelination in the brain occurs; there is a great deal of variability in cognitive functioning among patients with MS
    - Cognitive changes may occur in 30% to 70% of persons with MS (in some cases the cognitive problems may be quite minor, but for others the impairments can be severe)
    - Rudimentary or simple Attention is usually preserved although divided Attention and Mental Speed may be affected by the disorder

- Immediate Memory span typically remains intact as does Memory storage; the most common Memory deficit is with information retrieval or with the ability to spontaneously recall newly learned information out of storage (thus, recognition must also be assessed in Memory evaluations of patients with MS)
- With the exception of Dysarthria, language functions tend to remain relatively unaffected by the disease
- Tests of motor speed and coordination are most commonly impaired due to the effect of MS on motor and sensory functions
- In some patients with MS, deficits with planning, organization, and Problem Solving may occur

- Cognitive Rehabilitation should focus on helping the patient establish compensatory strategies to assist with impairments that most affect functional skills and independence, such as Memory and Problem Solving
- Patients and their families may benefit from counseling or support groups to help them deal with the disease (for a list of local support groups try the National Multiple Sclerosis Association of America [800–833–4MSA] or the National Multiple Sclerosis Society [212–463–7787])

Neglect. A patient's failure to respond to meaningful stimuli presented to the side contralateral to the cerebral lesion (also known as spatial inattention, hemi-inattention, visuospatial neglect, and unilateral spatial neglect).

- It is primarily a disorder of spatial Attention and *not* vision; patients fail to attend to the contralateral side of space because it no longer exists for them, they have no Awareness of that side of space
- Neglect is most common after Right Hemisphere lesions, particularly with damage to the Parietal Lobe, and occurs most frequently following Cerebrovascular Accidents (CVAs) or Tumors
- Neglect following a CVA usually occurs only after a larger stroke
- Patients may fail to attend to auditory, visual, and physical stimulation presented on the neglect side; presuming a Right Hemisphere CVA, they may only shave the right side of their face, eat food on the right side of their plates, dress the right side of their bodies, bump into objects on the left, be unaware of the left side of their bodies, and deviate their gaze continuously toward the right
- Neglect may or may not occur with hemiparesis; it is associated with impaired Constructional Ability and other disorders of Perceptual Functioning as well as denial of illness/deficits (Anosognosia)
- Neglect occurs in about one-third to one-half of Right Hemisphere CVAs
- It should not be confused with Hemianopsia, which affects the visual tracks but leaves spatial Attention intact; patients with neglect may also have a Visual Field Cut although the two disorders may exist independently and are not related neuroanatomically; Hemianopsia is easily compensated for but neglect is not (for example, if you close your left eye you are still aware that objects exist on your left side even though you can no longer see them, but patients with a left neglect lose that Awareness even though their vision is intact)

- Patients with neglect are often safety risks because they fail to appreciate hazards on their neglected side
- The probability of functional recovery decreases when neglect is present (due in part to the safety problems associated with the neglect itself but also due to the accompanying impairments of poor insight, the larger size of the CVA, and other cognitive impairments associated with Right Hemisphere damage)
- Recovery of neglect is variable; some studies have revealed a median recovery time of 9–26 weeks

Assessment of Neglect

- Qualitative observation of patients will provide insight about their visual gaze preference, their ability to maintain eye contact with you even when sitting on their non-neglected side, their ability to navigate without bumping into objects on their left, and their attention to all sides of space when eating, grooming, dressing, and bathing
- Line Bisection Tasks
- Cancellation Tests (assess where and how many target stimuli are missed as well as where the patient begins the search—most people without neglect should begin these tasks in the upper left hand corner, as if they are about to read)
- Drawing objects from Memory such as a clock and a daisy
- Copying objects such as a Greek cross
- Reading (does the patient scan all the way to the left-hand margin?)
- Double simultaneous stimulation (see Extinction)
- Monitor how well the patient responds to suggestions to look further to the left or if told that he or she missed some things on the left (if verbal cues do not increase left sided Attention, which they frequently do not, then other strategies will need to be used to facilitate Awareness of the neglected side)
- To assess insight and Awareness, ask patients if they are aware of any problems looking to the left or if they are aware of any changes with their vision

Treatment Suggestions for Left Neglect

- There is no single well-validated treatment for neglect that has been proven to work with all patients; treatment approaches should likely be varied with each patient and assessed as to their efficacy
- Increase Awareness and insight of patients regarding their neglect, how it affects their functioning and safety, how it is related to their brain injury, and what treatment will be offered
- Educate family members about the neglect syndrome and what they can do to help the patient
- Increase stimulation on the neglected side by interacting with patients at their midline (in cases of severe neglect) or in their neglected side of space
- Approach patients on their left; ask family and visitors to stand on the left side of the patient's bed when talking with him or her
- If possible, place the patient's bed in a position where more stimulation is on the left than the right side
- Place brightly colored objects, watches, bracelets, etc. on the patient's left arm or wrist to increase stimulation and awareness of the left
- Encourage patients to maintain eye contact during conversation
- Practice scanning and cancellation tasks; give patients concrete feedback about their performance; ask them how they can improve their own abilities in this area
- If using scanning tasks to increase left-sided attention, use stimuli that are intrinsically motivating for the patient (e.g., ask patients to scan for money scattered on a tabletop or for other objects important to them)
- Encourage patients to verbally self-cue aloud or to themselves to look further to the left
- Because patients with neglect cannot gauge internally how far they are scanning to their neglected side, try to

give them concrete or external markers to use as feedback for their scanning (e.g., suggest to patients that they turn their heads to the left until they see their left shoulder or until their chin touches their shoulder)

- Scanning can be facilitated by patients moving their left or right arm to the end of the area on the neglected side that is to be scanned
- To facilitate scanning while reading, place a bold colored line at the edge of the page and instruct the patient to scan to the left until they see the colored line
- Some research has found that patching the right eye for left neglect may benefit some patients while they are patched, although the long-term benefits of eye patching are unknown
- Incorporate activities that require scanning but that are interesting to the patient (e.g., incorporate scanning into a horticulture activity if the patient enjoys gardening or position the patient who is interested in sports in front of a television so that he or she must look to the left to watch an athletic contest)
- When placing objects (or yourself) in the neglected field, ensure that they are not placed so far to the left that the patient does not perceive them—the objects should be placed so that the patient must make an effort to see them but not so far as to make the task overly frustrating
- Before beginning a task or activity that requires scanning, ask the patient to first explore the enviroment visually and tactally to find the boundaries of the area to be explored; ask patients to explain what they are perceiving and how they know that they have found the boundaries
- Use multisensory stimulation, such as movement, sound, tactile, etc. on the left to increase Awareness
- Some authors have suggested that playing music for the patient may help activate the Right Hemisphere and improve neglect although this has not been demonstrated empirically

- As the neglect and scanning improve, objects can be placed further to the left and the complexity and demands on speed of mental processing can be increased

Chatterjee, A. (1995). Unilateral spatial neglect: Assessment and rehabilitation strategies. *NeuroRehabilitation, 5,* 115–128.

Hier, D. B., Mondlock, J., & Caplan, L. R. (1983). Behavioral abnormalities after right hemisphere stroke. *Neurology, 33,* 337–344.

Hier, D. B., Mondlock, J., & Caplan, L. R. (1983). Recovery of behavioral abnormalities after right hemisphere stroke. *Neurology, 33,* 345–350.

Neoplasm. See Tumor.

Neurobehavioural Rating Scale. A 27-item scale administered by clinicians to assess the behavioral sequelae of TBI; the items cover a wide range of potential behavioral, emotional, social, cognitive, and physical problems associated with brain injury; each item is rated on a 7-point scale from "not present" to "extremely severe"; the scale appears useful as a clinical and research tool in assessing outcome in TBI.

Corrigan, J. D., Dickerson, J., Fisher, E., & Meyer, P. (1990). The Neurobehavioural Rating Scale: Replication in an acute, inpatient rehabilitation setting. *Brain Injury, 4,* 215–222.

Levin, H. S., High, W. M., Goethe, K. E. et al. (1987). The Neurobehavioural Rating Scale: Assessment of the behavioural sequelae of head injury by the clinician. *Journal of Neurology, Neurosurgery, and Psychiatry, 50,* 183–193.

Neuropsychiatrist. A physician with specialized training and/or board certification in both psychiatry and neurology; the field of neuropsychiatry encompasses the study and treatment of psychiatric aspects of neurologic diseases and an approach to psychiatric disorders that emphasizes the role of brain dysfunction.

Normal Pressure Hydrocephalus (NPH). A condition that occurs in the elderly in which the Cerebrospinal Fluid (CSF) is inadequately reabsorbed by the brain resulting in enlarged Ventricles (Hyrocephalus) but without an increase in Intracranial Pressure (due to the shrinkage of brain tissue through Atrophy the cranial vault is able to accommodate the additional CSF); the most common triad of symptoms include Ataxia, urinary incontinence, and Dementia.

Nystagmus. Involuntary rhythmic horizontal, vertical, or rotary eyeball movements; may be caused by neurologic disorders including Multiple Sclerosis, damage to the Brain Stem, and alcohol/drug abuse.

Object Assembly. A subtest on the Wechsler Intelligence Scale for Children—III and the Wechsler Adult Intelligence Scale—Revised which measures Constructional Ability by requiring the subject to put together puzzle pieces under timed conditions; it is generally sensitive to right Posterior lesions.

Obsessive-Compulsive Disorder (OCD). A type of Anxiety disorder in which the person exhibits recurrent obsessions (intrusive and persistent ideas, thoughts, or impulses which cause Anxiety or distress, e.g., repeated thoughts about safety, contamination, the future) or compulsions (repetitive behaviors, e.g., hand washing, counting, checking doors or personal effects) which are severe enough to be time consuming or cause emotional distress; persons can have characteristics of OCD and not meet full criteria for the disorder, for example, the patient whose constant worrying interferes with rehabilitation; relaxation training and thought stopping techniques can be effective interventions for some patients.

Occipital Lobes. The most Posterior lobes of the cerebral Cortex; it is the location of the primary visual area (the Optic Nerves from the eyes terminate in the medial or interior portions of the occipital lobes); lesions to these brain structures may result in discrete blind spots in the corresponding visual fields (see Cortical Blindness), visual Agnosia, or other visual distortions (e.g., Balint's Syndrome, Prosopognosia, and Achromatopsia).

Oculomotor Nerve. Cranial Nerve III; one of the three Cranial Nerves (the other two being IV and VI) which move the eyes in unison to provide normal conjugate gaze; this nerve originates in the Midbrain and controls pupil constriction, the eyelid, and adductor and elevator muscles in each eye; lesions to the oculomotor nerve may lead to pupil dilatation, ptosis (drooping eyelid), and outward deviation of the eye.

Olfactory Hallucination. An Hallucination of smells that are not present; may be a manifestation of partial complex Seizures.

Olfactory Nerve. Cranial Nerve I; this nerve transmits the sensation of smell to the brain; because of its location on the undersurface of the Frontal Lobes, it can be sensitive to TBI (see Anosmia); a decreased sense of smell is also a normal Aging Effect.

Optic Nerve. Cranial Nerve II; these nerves convey visual information from the eye to the cerebral Cortex, specifically to the Occipital Lobes, and light intensity from the eye to the Brain Stem; damage to the optic nerve may result in Visual Field Cuts or Hemianopsia as well as a lack of pupillary constriction to light.

Orientation. Awareness of oneself and one's surroundings; the term oriented in three spheres (O×3) typically refers to patients' knowledge of their name (person), where they are (place), and the day, month, and year (time); may also refer to patients' knowledge of their reason for hospitalization (O×4).

- Orientation to person is least resistant to deterioration following brain insult or trauma
- Causes of disorientation include Delirium, Dementia, the acute effects of Traumatic Brain Injury and Posttraumatic Amnesia, and many other severe brain insults, particulary during the acute recovery period
- Orientation may not be able to be assessed in patients with Aphasia
- If patients are not fully oriented, they will likely have significant short-term Memory impairments; Autobiographical Memory and long-term Memory may also be significantly impaired
- Patients in Posttraumatic Amnesia following TBI are not oriented
- Patients may be fully oriented and still have Memory impairments (being fully oriented is a rather rudimenta-

ry function and should not be interpreted as a resumption of normal Memory)

- Patients who are disoriented following TBI most often (70%) become reoriented first to person, then place, then time; a smaller proportion (13%) become reoriented to time before place (High, Levin, & Gray, 1990)
- When disoriented to time, most patients provide a backward displacement of the date (e.g., give a year or month previous to the current one)
- In the majority of cases, patients must first become oriented before any attempt at rehabilitating short-term Memory deficits can begin
- The most common measure of orientation following TBI is the Galveston Orientation and Amnesia Test although informal assessment of orientation can be easily accomplished by asking orientation questions directly
- In assessing orientation, close approximations to the correct answers reflect better functioning than answers that differ substantially from the correct ones
- During recovery from TBI, orientation may fluctuate greatly during the day and may be affected by fatigue, medication effects, overstimulation, etc.
- Disorientation does not resolve suddenly or all at once; disorientation gradually resolves with time
- Patients who are disoriented are more likely to exhibit Agitation than those who are fully oriented

Treatment Suggestions for Disorientation

- Written orienting information must be easily available to the patient (use orientation signs or a Memory Log and include only the most basic information, e.g., month, year, place, reason for hospitalization, age, date of birth, and address if the latter are unknown by the patient)
- The more severely confused, the less information the patient should be given
- Reorient the patient first to autobiographical information and to the most important current orienting data (e.g., place and time)

- Reorient the patient only if it does not cause or increase Agitation
- Use recent pictures of family members, events, car, home, etc. to facilitate long-term Memory
- Engage patient in familiar hobbies, interests, TV, music, etc.
- Keep the patient's day structured, consistent, and predictable
- Try to avoid taking the patient off the rehabilitation unit
- Avoid room changes
- In some cases, family members can make audio or video tapes of orienting information which the patient can listen to or watch when not in therapy
- Each time you see the patient, identify yourself and your role
- Use labeled photographs of the patient's therapists to help orient the patient to the treatment team
- Reassure and calm the patient if frightened and confused
- See if patients can first answer orientation questions spontaneously before giving them the answer; determine how well they respond to cues such as multiple choices
- Keep in mind that disorientation is accompanied by Memory and attentional impairments so communication should be kept simple and brief
  - Give one command or instruction at a time
  - Do NOT give complex instructions
  - Do NOT expect patient to remember instructions or techniques
  - Orienting information should be given consistently across team members
  - Agree as a team what specific words will be told to the patient about his or her reason for hospitalization (see Awareness entry)
  - New learning at this stage may occur only through repeated and consistent practice
- Educate family members and visitors about the methods and reasons for these interventions; family members may need to become very involved with reorienting the patient as he or she may not believe the treatment staff

- See Rancho Los Amigos Cognitive Scale (Levels IV–VI) for additional suggestions

High, W. M., Levin, H. S., & Gray, H. E. (1990). Recovery of orientation following closed-head trauma. *Journal of Clinical and Experimental Neuropsychology, 12*, 703–714.

Paced Auditory Serial Addition Test (PASAT). A challenging measure of Mental Speed, Concentration, and divided Attention sensitive to the effects of Mild Traumatic Brain Injury.

Gronwall, D., & Wrightson, P. (1981). Memory and information processing capacity after closed head injury. *Journal of Neurology, Neurosurgery, and Psychiatry, 44*, 889–895.

Paraphasic Error. An error of verbal expression in which the person substitutes a sound (e.g., "bork" for fork) or a word of similar meaning (e.g., "spoon" for fork) for the intended word; a symptom of Aphasia.

Parietal Lobes. Bilateral cortical brain structures that lie Posterior to the Frontal and Temporal Lobes but Anterior to the Occipital Lobes; also referred to as the posterior association cortex; they are the site of integration of information involving sight, touch, body awareness, verbal comprehension, and logical/visuospatial relationships (i.e., comprehension of concepts such as "between" or "bigger and smaller").

- Lesions to the parietal lobes of either hemisphere may result in impaired Constructional Ability (although this is far more common in the Right Hemisphere), contralateral lower visual field deficits, contralateral Astereognosis, and misperception in the temporal order of when stimuli are presented
- Left parietal lobe damage may result in fluent Aphasia, Echolalia, Alexia (inability to read), Agraphia (inability to write), Apraxia, and Acalculia
- Right parietal lobe lesions may produce impairments with Constructional Ability, spatial Acalculia, dressing Apraxia, Neglect (left sided), and Anosognosia and decreased Awareness of deficits

Lezak, M. D. (1995). Neuropsychological assessment (3rd ed.). New York: Oxford University Press.

Parkinson's Disease (PD). A progressive disorder in which there is a gradual degeneration of the substantia nigra (part of the motor system of the Basal Ganglia) which results in substantially reduced production of the neurotransmitter dopamine.

- PD can be caused by repeated head trauma and toxic and viral exposure although the etiology for most cases in unknown
- The most common features of PD are motor problems including resting tremors which can affect limbs, jaws/face, and trunk, problems initiating movements, motor slowing (Bradykinesia), shuffling gait, and blank facial expressions (masked facies)
- Depression is common among persons with PD
- Estimates vary although the incidence of Dementia in PD has been reported as between 10%–40%; cognitive problems may be absent, or range from mild to severe
- When the onset of PD is before the ages of 40 or 45, there tend to be a slower rate of progression and fewer cognitive problems; with onset after age 70, the rates of Dementia increase rapidly
- With increased Bradykinesia and physical rigidity, cognitive impairments tend to be most pronounced; when tremor is the most prominent physical symptom, cognitive problems tend to be milder
    - Cognitive impairments can be similar to those found in patients with Frontal Lobe disorders due to the interconnections between the subcortical structures involved with PD and frontal brain structures
    - Mental slowing (Bradyphrenia) is common as well as problems with sustained and shifting Attention
    - Rate of learning is usually slowed and delayed recall or retrieval of information is likely to be impaired (cueing and recognition, however, usually normalizes performance)
    - Dysarthria and micrographia (small writing) are common although most language functions remain intact
    - Higher level Problem Solving and conceptual functioning may be compromised due to difficulty with cognitive rigidity and in formulating Problem Solving strategies

- When treating patients with cognitive impairments, speak slowly, allow patients time to process information, treat in a distraction-free environment if possible, don't shift topics quickly, and provide patients with cues or prompts to recall newly learned information
- Persons with PD often have discrete periods when their functioning is better than at other times; rehabilitation may help patients and their families recognize these "on/off" times and how to maximize functioning around them
- Cognitive Rehabilitation can assist patients to learn to compensate for their cognitive weaknesses
- Patients and families may benefit from support groups to assist with Adjustment to the illness and disability (for local support groups call the National Parkinson Foundation [800–327–4545])

Lezak, M. D. (1995). *Neuropsychological assessment* (3rd ed.). New York: Oxford University Press.

Perceptual Functioning. A nonspecific term used to describe the manner in which sensory information is perceived by the individual; it may refer to the perception of auditory, tactile, or olfactory information although it is most often associated with the perception of visual stimuli (i.e., visual-perceptual or visuoperceptual functioning).

Types of Visual Perceptual Functioning

- Inattention or Neglect
- Visual scanning
- Constructional Ability
- Perception of angulation: the ability to judge angles of varying degrees (see Judgment of Line Orientation Test)
- Facial recognition (see Facial Recognition Test and Prosopognosia)
- Visual organization: the ability to recognize or create percepts out of ambiguous, incomplete, or fragmented visual stimuli; this includes the concept of visual closure in which the patient is asked to identify an object based on a partial drawing or representation of it (see Hooper Visual Organization Test, Object Assembly Subtest)

- Visual interference: the ability to perceive or recognize complete objects or pictures when they are masked by extraneous lines or designs; assessment of this function would include the use of figure-ground tests and overlapping and embedded figures (e.g., Hidden Figures Test and Overlapping Figures Test)

Lezak, M. D. (1995). *Neuropsychological assessment* (3rd ed.). New York: Oxford University Press.

Perseveration. The continuation of an activity or a response after it is no longer appropriate; it reflects the inability to shift responses or to stop responding after the cessation of the causative stimulus; perseveration may occur verbally (e.g., repeating the same word over and over again) or motorically (e.g., performing the same motor act over and over again).

Suggested Subtypes of Perseveration

- *Recurrent Perseveration*: The unintentional repetition, after cessation, of a previously emitted response to a subsequent stimulus (e.g., when asked to name objects, the patient provides the name of an object presented earlier); this is most common in patients with Aphasia and Dementia
- *Stuck-in-set Perseveration*: The inappropriate maintenance of a current category or framework (e.g., after having recited the days of the week in *backward* order, the patient has difficulty counting *forward* from 1 to 20 because he or she keeps reverting to counting backward or after combing his hair, the patient is given a toothbrush and he attempts to apply it to his hair); this is most common with impaired Executive Functioning and with lesions to the Frontal Lobes
- *Continuous Perseveration*: The inappropriate repetition, without interruption, of a current behavior; this may be more obvious with motor behavior (e.g., when asked to draw a circle, the patient keeps drawing them until told to stop, or during ADLs the patient has to be told when to stop washing her one body part and to move on to another one); this may be more common in patients with lesions to Subcortical Structures or the Frontal Lobes (see Executive Functioning)

Assessment of Perseveration

- Observe patients perform their usual daily activities and monitor their ability to shift their behavior and terminate responses appropriately
- Monitor perseveration in patients' verbal and motor responses as well as their ideas and the content of their conversations
- Informal tasks such as asking patients to draw repetitive patterns (e.g., the pattern "++0++0++0" or alternating but connecting m's and n's in cursive writing) can assess perseveration
- Formal tests such as the Wisconsin Card Sorting Test, Category Test, and Trail Making Test can also be sensitive to perseverative responses

Treatment Suggestions for Perseveration

- There is no single, well-validated treatment for perseveration due to its association with significant brain injury (i.e., it often reflects substantial brain damage and is usually accompanied by multiple cognitive deficits)
- The patient may require hand-on-hand interventions to stop a perseverative response as he or she may not respond to verbal commands or instructions
- Make a "clean break" or pause a few minutes between activities or tasks to decrease the likelihood of a perseverative response
- After completing an activity, try a different task that is completely unrelated to the previous one; patients may tend to perseverate more among tasks that are somewhat similar than if they are different
- Try to have patients self-verbalize or self-talk when to shift from one activity to another
- See if patients will repond to an external stimulus, such as counting to 10 or watching a timer, to cue them to stop or shift tasks

Sandson, J., & Albert, M. L. (1984). Varieties of perseveration. *Neuropsychologia, 22*, 715–732.

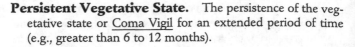

Persistent Vegetative State. The persistence of the vegetative state or Coma Vigil for an extended period of time (e.g., greater than 6 to 12 months).

Personality. An enduring pattern of how one perceives, relates to, or thinks about oneself, others, and the world; premorbid personality affects how a person may respond or adjust to his or her disability and rehabilitation treatment; neurologic disorders, such as Seizures, Dementia, brain Tumors, Cerebrovascular Accidents, and Multiple Sclerosis can also affect personality; in moderate to severe Traumatic Brain Injury, personality is often affected (the most common changes are irritability and self-centeredness); see also Frontal Lobes, Executive Functioning, and Personality Disorder.

Personality Disorder. An enduring pattern of inner experience and behavior that deviates markedly from others in the same culture, is generally inflexible over time, has an onset by early adulthood, and leads to distress, impairment, or maladaptive relationships between the person and others.

- Personality disorders (and traits) can greatly affect a person's response to and ability to benefit from rehabilitation
- Personality factors often influence interpersonal relationships between the patient and staff as well as the patient's adaptation to change, stress, lack of control, and the disabling condition
- Personality can also be affected by brain damage itself and can be changed, in some cases significantly, by Traumatic Brain Injury
- If brain injury has altered personality functioning, then personality and behavior problems can be part of treatment, but if personality difficulties existed premorbidly, then rehabilitation will not change those behaviors
- Dealing with individuals in rehabilitation whose personality interferes with treatment requires close coordination of treatment interventions and very consistent approaches to the patient

- For patients with personality problems, expectations and consequences of behavior need to be specific, concrete, and consistently applied by all treating therapists
- Ask family members for advice on how to deal more effectively with the patient and enlist their aid in increasing cooperation from the patient
- See Behavior Contracts, Behavior Management, and Motivation entries for further suggestions

Some Personality Disorder Subtypes (from DSM IV)

- *Paranoid*: Distrustful and suspicious of others' motives
- *Schizoid*: Detached from social relationships
- *Antisocial*: Disregards the rights of others
- *Borderline*: Instable in interpersonal relationships, self-image, and Affect
- *Histrionic*: Excessively emotional and attention seeking
- *Avoidant*: Socially inhibited and hypersensitive to criticism
- *Narcissistic*: Grandiose and in need of admiration but lacks empathy for others
- *Dependent*: Submissive and needing to be taken care of
- *Obsessive-Compulsive*: Preoccupied with orderliness, perfectionism, and control

Photophobia. An increased sensitivity to light; may result from Mild Traumatic Brain Injury.

Pia Mater. A thin connective tissue membrane closest to the brain that carries blood vessels; it covers and adheres to the brain surface and extends into the sulci; it is the innermost of the three membranes covering the brain; see also Arachnoid, Dura Mater, and Meninges.

Pick's Disease. A progressive Dementia that results in degeneration of Anterior brain structures, particularly the Frontal Lobes; Frontal Lobe degeneration usually causes marked Personality changes and disinhibited behaviors even before cognitive deficits are readily apparent; Pick's Disease usually develops before age 65; it is an uncommon form of Dementia.

Picture Arrangement. A subtest from the Wechsler Intelligence Scale for Children—III and the Wechsler Adult Intelligence Scale—Revised that requires the person to rearrange a series of cartoon-like pictures to make the most sensible story; it is sensitive to Right Hemisphere and diffuse brain damage.

Picture Completion. A subtest from the Wechsler Intelligence Scale for Children—III and the Wechsler Adult Intelligence Scale—Revised that requires the person to identify what important part is missing from a series of incomplete pictures; it is a measure of visual recognition and Perceptual Functioning but also requires some reasoning, remote Memory, and general information.

Pons. Located above the Medulla in the Brain Stem, the Pons assists with postural and muscle movements; it refines and regulates motor impulses; the Pons contains substantial motor pathways between the Cerebrum and the Cerebellum; damage to the Pons may cause problems with motor functioning and Cranial Nerve involvement although cognitive functions should be relatively spared.

Portland Adaptability Inventory (PAI). A set of three scales (Temperament and Emotionality, Abilities and Social Relationships, Physical Relationships) constructed to provide a systematic record of the personal and social maladaptations of head trauma patients; there are a total of 24 items on which the patient is rated by a clinician on a scale of 0 (no problem) to 3 (severe problems); ratings can be based on patient/family reports, observations, records, and social history.

Lezak, M. D. (1987). Relationships between personality disorders, social disturbances, and physical disability following brain injury. *Journal of Head Trauma Rehabilitation, 2*, 57–69.

Positron Emission Tomography (PET scan). A functional neuroimaging technique in which cerebral blood flow and volume and regional glucose metabolism are studied to evaluate cerebral physiology; this technique has been used in the study of both neurologic and psychiatric illnesses although it is a very expensive procedure and unavailable in most medical settings; there is a small body of knowledge regarding its usefulness in a TBI population, suggesting that it may be more sensitive than some other neuroimaging techniques to brain damage; see also Single Photon Emission Computed Tomograpy (SPECT).

Postconcussive Syndrome. A constellation of vague and often nonspecific physical, cognitive, and affective symptoms following Mild Traumatic Brain Injury; problems with Memory, Concentration, and headache are often reported; may also be known as posttraumatic head injury syndrome; see Mild Traumatic Brain Injury entry.

Posterior. The back surface; behind or after.

Posterior Cerebral Artery (PCA). The PCA is one of the three main sources of blood supply to the brain, it branches from the Basilar Artery off the Circle of Willis and sends branches to the middle and lower surfaces of the Temporal Lobes and to the middle portion of the Occipital Lobes; lesions to the PCA may result in Hemianopsia and other Visual Field Cuts, Memory disorders, some aphasic symptoms (on the left) and perceptual disturbances (on the right); see also Cerebral Circulation.

Posttraumatic Amnesia (PTA). A period of Amnesia and disorientation following Traumatic Brain Injury.

- PTA may be very brief and last only seconds or may extend for weeks to months
- It is a very important measure of injury severity (i.e., the longer the period of PTA the more severe the injury)
  - PTA less than 24 hours is associated with mild brain injury
  - PTA from 1 to 7 days is associated with moderate brain injury
  - PTA greater than 7 days is associated with severe brain injury

- PTA may occur with or without Coma but it is longer and more extensive if it follows a loss of consciousness
- PTA of greater than 7 days has been associated with Memory impairment in more than half of patients studied; PTA of greater than 2 weeks has been associated with poor outcome and a high level of burden on family members of the TBI survivor; PTA greater than 4 weeks is strongly associated with severe disability and an inability to return to work
- During PTA, patients may be agitated and are often inattentive and highly distractible; they are often sensitive to overstimulation and may exhibit long-term or Autobiographical Memory deficits (in addition to short-term Memory problems) during this period
- Assessment of higher cognitive functions should be deferred until the resolution of PTA
- Measurement of PTA can be done informally by asking rudimentary mental status questions or by formal and more standardized instruments such as the Galveston Orientation and Amnesia Test (a score of 75 or greater on two successive days is considered an indication that PTA has resolved) or the Ross Information Processing Assessment
- PTA resolves gradually; the level of disorientation and confusion may fluctuate from day to day or even hourly
- Unlike Retrograde Amnesia, the length of Amnesia following the resolution of PTA does not "shrink" (i.e., after PTA resolves, patients will not recall events that occurred during that time)
- During PTA, focus on reorienting the patient, managing behavior and Agitation (if the latter is present), structuring the patient's environment, and emphasizing functional/overlearned tasks
- For treatment suggestions for patients in PTA please refer to the following entries: Agitation, Attention, Memory, Orientation, and Rancho Los Amigos Cognitive Scale (Levels IV–VI)
- Figure 7 depicts the relationship among Retrograde Amnesia, Coma, and PTA

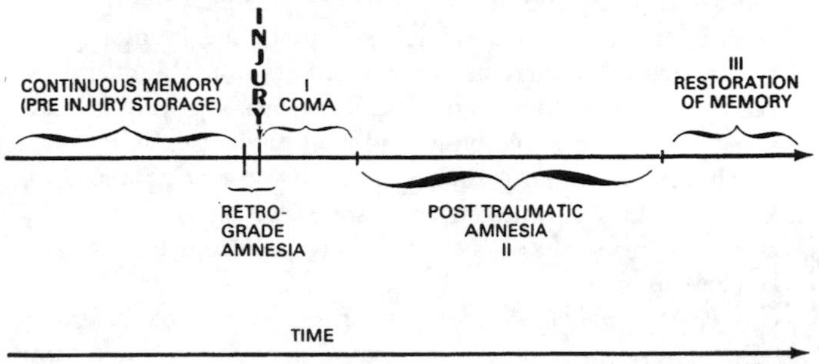

Figure 7. Sequence of alterations in memory after closed head injury. The periods of coma (I) and posttraumatic amnesia (II) have traditionally been combined to yield a total interval of impaired consciousness that extends until continuous memory for ongoing events (III) is established. (Reprinted with permission of authors from *Neurobehavioral Consequences of Closed Head Injury* by H. S. Levin, A. L. Benton, and R. G. Grossman, 1982, p. 74. Copyright 1982 by Oxford University Press, Inc.)

Posttraumatic Stress Disorder (PTSD). A psychiatric disorder that may develop following exposure to an extreme traumatic stressor such as the threat of death or serious injury to oneself or others; the symptoms broadly include a reexperiencing of the trauma in dreams, flashbacks, etc., a persistent avoidance of stimuli associated with the trauma, numbing of general emotional responsiveness, and persistent symptoms of increased Arousal.

Problem Solving. A complex ability closely related to Abstract and Conceptual Thinking (the boundaries between all of these concepts are somewhat arbitrary) that involves the processing of information and situations to produce and execute viable solutions to tasks that need to be accomplished; problem solving skills are applicable to a wide range of activities and are required for very simple tasks, such as sequencing one's morning routine, and for very complex interactions, such as how to look for a job; although the Frontal Lobes and Executive Functions are related to this ability, it is a complex and multifaceted mental process that requires the integration of multiple brain and cognitive systems.

- There is no unitary theory of problem solving and decision making although there is some conceptual agreement among researchers as to the necessary steps for effective problem solving:
  - *Problem identification*: Patients must be able to accurately identify that a problem exists, that they may have some role in the creation of the problem and in generating possible solutions to the problem, and a willingness to correct the problem
  - *Production of possible solutions*: In this phase, patients need to generate possible solutions to the problem and to evaluate or assess their potential effectiveness; a plan or solution must be decided upon
  - *Application of the solution*: At this stage, patients must act on or execute the plan to solve the problem
  - *Evlauating the outcome*: The patient must determine if the problem was solved adequately or if further modifications or solutions are necessary
- Impaired problem solving can be the result of deficits from one of a number of cognitive areas
- Problem solving deficits can be subtle and affect functioning in very limited ways or they can severely impair an individual's capabilities to perform even simple daily tasks
- Problem solving skills are likely multidimensional, meaning that different skills and abilities are necessary to solve different types of problems effectively (i.e., there is not likely a single "problem solving ability" but rather many different abilities that can be applied to many different types of problems); as a result, a patient may be unable to solve one type of problem but can easily solve others

- Increasing age can adversely affect problem solving skills (see Age Effects entry)
- Emotional factors, such as Depression, Anxiety, and Motivation, can affect problem solving

Cognitive Deficits That Can Alter Problem Solving Skills

- One of the major impediments to effective problem solving is Impulsivity; impulsive responses do not allow patients to think carefully about problems or to generate multiple possible solutions and their consequences
- Decreased Awareness that problems exist, of the patient's role in contributing to the problem, and of the patient's responsibility in generating possible solutions
- A lack of drive (known as Abulia in severe cases) which may limit patients' ability to execute plans or to apply problem solving strategies
- Impaired Attention, Memory, or Perceptual Functioning; patients in Delirium, Posttraumatic Amnesia, or other confusional state will exhibit limited problem solving skills
- A lack of knowledge in a specific area will obviously hinder a person's ability to solve problems efficiently in that domain
- Impaired reasoning, Abstract Thinking, and cognitive flexibility (i.e., the inability to generate more than one solution to a problem or to think of a problem in only one way) will limit problem solving efficiency; Concrete Thinking interferes with problem solving and decision making

Assessment of Problem Solving Skills

- Determine patients' premorbid problem solving capabilities; some patients with TBI will have a history of poor judgment and impulsive decision making which will need to be considered in setting goals for treatment and in establishing interventions in this area
- Observe patients as they attempt to solve pragmatic, everyday problems and assess how they respond to minor challenges and complications

- In order to assess problem solving competence with a specific task (e.g., dialing 911 or taking medication on time), try to test the patient's ability to perform that specific task under conditions that resemble the environment in which the problem solving behavior is to be exhibited (as much as possible)
- Do not expect patients' self-report of their judgment and problem solving skills to be accurate, as persons tend to overestimate their competence in performing many tasks
- Assess patients' general cognitive abilities such as their Memory, Attention, Mental Speed, language, and Perceptual Functioning, as significant deficits in these areas can adversely affect problem solving skills
- Ask patients questions about what they would do under specific circumstances or with specific problems such as if they locked themselves out of their house, if they forgot to take their medication over a few days, etc.
- When appropriate norms are available, use tests of Abstract and Conceptual Thinking such as the Similarities and Comprehension subtests of the Wechsler Adult Intelligence Scale—Revised, the Wisconsin Card Sorting Test, Category Test, etc.; as with general cognitive skills, an adequate performance on these measures tends to provide evidence of necessary but not always sufficient problem solving skills
- Examine the patient's Awareness of his or her deficits and how these deficits may affect safety and judgment

Treatment Suggestions for Problem Solving Deficits

- It is very difficult to remediate general impairments with reasoning and judgment; in patients with these deficits, it is best to teach compensatory techniques or domain-specific skills (e.g., teach or practice specific skills for specific problems)
- Problem solving and reasoning skills do not easily generalize to situations outside of treatment, so a focus on how to solve a specific problem in the patient's own environment will likely be more effective

- If impairments with Memory, Attention, and other cognitive functions are evident, then ongoing Cognitive Rehabilitation for these deficits would be appropriate and may help to improve problem solving somewhat
- Improve patients' Awareness of their impairments, how they affect their safety and functioning, and what they need to do to compensate for them
- Use reasoning exercises (there are, for example, several workbooks available that provide exercises for patients to practice convergent and divergent thinking, inductive reasoning, etc.), however, recognize that these interventions do not generalize well to problems outside of therapy and that their main benefits may be to help patients become more aware of their limitations and to provide a forum to discuss their problem solving strategies
- If difficulties with decreased drive interfere with the execution of problem solving strategies, then address that deficit directly (see Abulia for treatment suggestions)
- Teach patients a process or give them a model or template to solve their problems (i.e., teach them the steps about how they should go about trying to solve their problems in a deliberate and methodical manner)
- Instruct patients in the SOLVE mnemonic
  - (S)pecify the problem to be solved
  - (O)ptions need to be generated and listed
  - (L)isten to others' advice
  - (V)alue clarification—decide what is most important
  - (E)valuate the results and refine the solutions as necessary
- Another decision making method is:
  - Gather information and list all possible options or solutions
  - List the advantages of each option
  - List the disadvantages of each option
  - Rate the emotional reaction related to each option
  - Make the decision
- Generate "What would happen if" conversations; encourage patients to always ask "What would happen if" before

they attempt a course of action or before they attempt to solve a complex problem (this can help patients recognize the consequences of their actions before they attempt solutions)

- If problems are noted with social judgment and behavior, then Social Skills Training may be appropriate
- Teach impulsive patients to slow down before making complex decisions (see Impulsivity); see if they will agree to wait a specific period of time before making important decisions
- See Executive Functions entry for additional treatment suggestions

Diehl, M., Willis, S. L., & Schaie, K. W. (1995). Everday problem solving in older adults: Observational assessment and cognitive correlates. *Psychology and Aging, 10,* 478–491.

Parente, R. (1995). *Executive functions: Rehabilitation strategies you can really use.* Lecture presented at the Eighth Annual Traumatic Brain Injury Seminar, Newport, RI.

Sohlberg, M. M., & Mateer, C. A. (1989). *Introduction to cognitive rehabilitation: Theory and practice.* New York: The Guilford Press.

Procedural Learning. Skill or motor learning; the ability to learn new techniques or procedures through consistent practice in spite of Amnesia for ongoing events and even though the patient cannot tell you verbally how to perform the task; see Memory.

Prosody. The tone and inflection of speech that conveys emotional or affective information, such as sadness, anger, joy, sarcasm, etc., beyond the meaning of the words alone; a lack of prosody (Aprosodia) may be evident in patients' expressive speech and in their ability to appreciate prosody in the speech of others; decreased prosody is most often present in Aphasia, particularly expressive or Broca's Aphasia, and in damage to the Right Hemisphere.

Prosopognosia. The inability to recognize previously known human faces or to learn new ones; patients can recognize others based on other characteristics such as voice, posture, clothing, etc.; patients with prosopognosia are able to recognize objects in their environment although they are unable to determine whether the specific object belongs to them or not; patients are able to identify the class to which objects belong (e.g., an automobile) although they may be unable to identify the specific member within that class (e.g., the manufacturer or type of car); prosopognosia is relatively rare and typically requires bilateral damage to the Occiptal and Parietal Lobes (most commonly due to Cerebrovascular Accident).

Pseudobulbar Affect. Rapid changes in Affect, for example, the person suddenly begins laughing or crying (the latter is more common), but without any change in Mood or emotions; i.e., the patient may suddenly become tearful when discussing his or her family but denies feelings of sadness or Depression; when the conversation changes to a neutral topic, the person's Affect returns to normal; some clinicians refer to this state as labile Affect, regardless of the internal feeling state of the individual, whereas others may refer to any Lability as a pseudobulbar state; it can be associated with structural lesions from stroke, Dementia, trauma, Multiple Sclerosis or any disorder that disrupts the frontal cortex and its connecting pathways to lower brain structures.

Treatment of Pseudobulbar Affect

- Educate patient and family about the effects of brain injury on emotional functioning and Lability
- Do not presume the patient is Depressed because of a rapid onset of tearfulness; inquire directly about Mood and feelings of sadness
- If the patient is not Depressed but frequently becomes tearful, keep conversations on neutral (nonemotional) topics
- Do not dwell on the patient's Affect
- Some antidepressant medications may be helpful
- A Pathological Laughing and Crying Scale has been developed which may help quantify the effects of treatment

Bishop, D. S., & Pet, R. (1995). Psychobehavioral problems other than depression in stroke. *Topics in Stroke Rehabilitation, 2*, 56–68.

Robinson, R. G., Parikh, R. M., Lipsey, J. R., Starkstein, S. E., & Price, T. R. (1993). Pathological laughing and crying following stroke: Validation of a measurement scale and a double-blind treatment study. *American Journal of Psychiatry, 150*, 286–293.

Pseudodementia. The appearance of Dementia (e.g., impaired cognitive functioning with a decline from prior levels presumed due to a biological or medical condition) but due to an underlying psychiatric disorder, most commonly Depression; that is, patients appear to be demented but are actually depressed (severe Depression in the elderly can significantly alter cognitive functioning); the Dementia is reversible if the Depression resolves.

Pseudoseizures. Seizure behavior, such as altered sensorium or motor signs of Seizures that are due to psychological causes; persons may have pseudoseizures in combination with epileptic seizures or other central nervous system disorders; also known as psychogenic Seizures; see Seizure entry.

Psychosis. An broadly defined term in psychiatry that typically refers to a condition in which Hallucinations and Delusions are prominent; psychosis is usually associated with Schizophrenia and Mania although neurologic disorders can also be a cause; psychosis has been known to occur with such disorders as Dementia, Seizures, metabolic encephalopathies, severe Traumatic Brain Injury, and Cerebrovascular Accidents, particularly those involving the Right Hemisphere.

Peroutka, S. J., Sohmer, B. H., Kumar, A. J., Folstein, M., & Robinson, R. G. (1982). Hallucinations and delusions following a right temporoparietal infarction. *The Johns Hopkins Medical Journal, 151*, 181–185.

Rancho Los Amigos Cognitive Scale. A guideline of eight levels of cognitive and behavioral recovery following Traumatic Brain Injury.

- The Rancho scale is helpful for designing treatment plans, understanding behavior, predicting progress, and helping the family to appreciate the patient's current/future needs
- The scale is meant only as a prospective guide; all patients do not pass through all eight levels (some patients skip levels, plateau at others, and even return to previous ones)
- Levels I to III are Coma levels; IV to VI are associated with Posttraumatic Amnesia; levels VII and VIII tend to be associated with postacute or community reentry rehabilitation

Ranchos Los Amigos Levels and Suggested Interventions

- NO RESPONSE (Level I): Patient appears to be in a deep sleep (Coma) and is completely unresponsive to stimuli
  Treatment Suggestions for Level I
  - Speak directly to the patient
  - Gently touch, stroke, and massage patient
  - Play patient's favorite music and TV programs
  - Audio or video tape record messages from friends and family and play for the patient
  - Establish contact with the family and begin to educate them on sequelae to brain injury
  - Refer family to national brain injury association and local chapters (telephone: 1–800–444–NHIF)

  Potential Assessment Measures for Level I
  - Glasgow Coma Scale
- GENERALIZED RESPONSE (Level II): Patient reacts inconsistently and nonpurposefully to stimuli in a nonspecific manner; responses may be physiological changes, gross body movements and/or vocalizations; responses are likely to be delayed
- LOCALIZED RESPONSE (Level III): Patient reacts specifically but inconsistently to stimuli; responses are directly related to the type of stimulus presented, as in turning the

head toward a sound or pushing away a painful stimulus; patient may follow simple commands in an inconsistent and delayed manner such as closing eyes or squeezing a hand; patient may respond to discomfort by pulling at nasogastric tubes and resisting restraints

Treatment Suggestions for Levels II and III

- The general cognitive goals at these levels are to prevent sensory deprivation and to increase responsivity of any type
- Continue education and support of the family
- Short but frequent interactions with the patient are preferable to long but infrequent sessions
- Place visually stimulating objects around the room and the patient's bedside such as colorful, familiar objects and pictures
- Television and music may be played intermittently but not continually as this tends to then become just background noise
- Attempt to place your own face in the patient's line of vision and become overexpressive with Affect
- Try to engage patients in fixing their visual gaze on an object or in tracking objects if only for a few seconds (this is an elementary way to begin assessing and treating rudimentary attentional functions)
- Use the patient's name and speak directly to him or her
- Orient the patient frequently
- Touch and stroke the patient gently
- Use different textures of wash clothes when bathing patient
- Provide oral stimulation by using flavored cleansing agents
- Use range of motion exercises and change bed position frequently
- Sit patient up if possible
- Attempt to channel any motor movement or response into a meaningful activity such as simple self-care

- Encourage the following of simple commands such as reaching, pulling, pointing, and tugging
- Consider the results of the patient's CT scan and type of injury when assessing his or her responses (e.g., if left Temporal Lobe damage is evident then the patient may be aphasic and unable to follow commands or if Right Hemisphere lesions are noted then a left Neglect may exist which would require approaching the patient on his right side to optimize stimulation)

Potential Assessment Measures for Levels II and III

- Glasgow Coma Scale
- Western Neuro Sensory Stimulation Profile
- Disability Rating Scale
- Individually tailored behavioral assessments designed to assess reactivity to external stimuli including responses to commands, simple inhibition, rudimentary visual tracking, and sustained visual or auditory Attention

- CONFUSED-AGITATED (Level IV): Patient is in a heightened state of activity with severely decreased ability to process information; behavior may be bizarre, nonpurposeful, and aggressive/agitated (Agitation occurs in approximately one third to one half of moderate to severe TBI patients); patient is amnestic (still in Posttraumatic Amnesia) and globally confused; very susceptible to overstimulation; patient requires help for self-care; elopement risk may be high; the patient has no insight or Awareness about his or her deficits; the patient's tolerance for pain and discomfort is very low and will escalate Agitation; see Agitation entry for further descriptions and treatment suggestions

Treatment Suggestions for Level IV

- The overall treatment goals are to decrease Agitation, increase Attention to the environment and rudimentary self-care skills, patient safety, and increase Orientation
- Educate families about the patient's level of internal confusion and disorganization; stress that the patient is

not responsible for his or her behavior and that there will be no Memory of this stage for the patient after it has cleared; inform family members that entry into this stage is a sign of progress

- Family visits may need to be modified; family may need to stay with the patient on a 24-hour basis or visits with family may need to be limited to certain members or at certain times depending on the patient's needs and how he or she responds behaviorally to family visits
- Educate all visitors about how to interact with the patient during this stage
- Limit visitors as appropriate
- Staff must be consistent in their approach to the patient and how the patient's behavior will be managed
- Keep the patient's daily schedule as consistent from day to day as possible
- If possible, elimiate the environmental stimuli and activities that are contributing to the Agitation
- Avoid loud noises and confusion in the patient's immediate enviroment
- Use medication sparingly
- Avoid physical restraints as this tends to increase Agitation
- Orient patients with signs, calendars, labeled pictures of family and therapists, etc. (see Memory and Memory Log)
- Place a large printed sign with the patient's first name on the door to his or her room
- Use the same words and rationale to the patient to describe why he or she is in the hospital (see Awareness)
- Keep language and verbal instructions brief and simple; try to keep sentences to less than 8–10 words
- Use soothing voice; stay in control
- Always identify yourself to the patient and what you are going to be doing with him or her
- Do not scold or show anger toward the patient

- Reassure patients of their safety, that they are in a good place, that their family knows where they are, and that their family wants them there
- Allow patient to see others in treatment
- Allow freedom of movement when possible but avoid taking the patient off the unit as this may increase confusion and elopement risk
- If you are doing something that is increasing the patient's Agitation, then STOP IT
- Use quiet treatment areas if available
- Be flexible and creative when dealing with patients in this stage; what worked yesterday may not work today
- Use distraction to avert or decrease Agitation (e.g., try to engage patient in another task or in a different conversation to de-escalate Agitation)
- Use automatic and familiar gross motor activities, such as ball throwing during this stage
- Try to engage the patient in his or her premorbid interests or hobbies if possible (and if cognitively able)
- Play the patient's favorite music, TV programs, etc.
- Remember that tolerance to one person may be very limited; staff may need to "switch off" the patient to another staff member if one person is not making progress; consider a staff member of a different age or gender

Potential Assessment Measures for Level IV

- Disability Rating Scale
- Functional Independence Measure and the Functional Assessment Measure
- Neurobehavioral Rating Scale
- Galveston Orientation and Amnesia Test
- Agitated Behavior Scale
- Rudimentary measures of Attention/Concentration, language functions (auditory comprehension and reading), task persistence, Orientation, and Perceptual Functioning

- CONFUSED-INAPPROPRIATE-NONAGITATED (Level V): Patient appears able to respond to simple commands with more consistency; responses can still be nonpurposeful and random; behavior is inappropriate and perhaps restless but not agitated; patient has gross Attention to the environment but is highly distractible; Memory remains severely impaired; patient is still in Posttraumatic Amnesia; insight and Awareness into deficits are lacking; tolerance for pain and discomfort is increasing although painful or noxious stimuli may increase restlessness and inappropriate behavior; ADLs still require guidance and structure; patient may still be a high elopement risk
- CONFUSED-APPROPRIATE (Level VI): Patient exhibits goal-directed behavior but is dependent on external input for direction; patient is able to tolerate discomfort with explanation from staff; patient follows simple directions consistently and shows carry-over for tasks that have been relearned, such as ADLs; new learning and Memory are impaired although the patient exhibits "islands" of recall for some recent events; some Awareness and insight are beginning to emerge; Orientation is improving (Posttraumatic Amnesia is resolving)

  Treatment Suggestions for Levels V and VI

  - Overall goals at these stages are to decrease cognitive confusion stemming from environmental sources, to increase cognitive abilities in a hierarchial sequence, and to increase Awareness and insight about the patient's current circumstances
  - Continue with family education about recovery from TBI and how the family should interact with the patient
  - Observe how family members interact with the patient and their tolerance for the Personality and cognitive changes exhibited by their loved one
  - Keep environment structured and predictable (e.g., have the same treatment sessions at the same time each day, consistent nursing staff)

- Provide organization to the patient that he or she may be unable to generate internally (e.g., assist with organizing and sequencing ADLs)
- Continue with Orientation activities but give fewer cues as the patient improves and becomes less confused
- Provide a Memory Log and other environmental cues to improve Orientation as appropriate (establish extent of Retrograde Amnesia and provide the patient with personal information to reestablish Autobiographical Memory)
- Place familiar and comforting objects and pictures within easy view of the patient
- Ask family to bring in recent pictures of family members or events labeled with the names and relationship of the person to the patient to review with him or her
- Continue to control environmental stimulation
- Place the patient's first name on the door to his or her room in large printed letters
- Use activities that are designed to increase sustained Attention and appropriate interaction with the others
- Attempt to engage patients in recreational activities that are familiar and of interest to them
- Provide patients with verbal/social praise and encouragement for their hard work
- Remain optimistic and positive for further recovery
- Orienting and treating in group sessions may now be possible
- Have patients write down and refer to their daily schedule if possible
- Gradually eliminate verbal cues as much as possible during routine care and attempt to have the patient rely more on *written* cues and reminders, such as lists and index cards (this gives patients more responsibility for their functioning and may decrease their need to have others present during some self-care activities)
- Monitor patients' behavioral and social functioning (e.g., appropriate social interaction, adequate behav-

ioral controls, and frustration tolerance); redirect patient as appropriate, give concrete feedback about inappropriate behaviors, increase insight about how others are reacting to patient, and instruct patient in rudimentary social skills (for very confused patients, verbal exchanges should be brief and will not be retained or remembered by the patient)

- Generally, the more confused the patient, the greater the likelihood of inappropriate behavior; patients who are very confused will not respond to logical arguments or long explanations about how they should act, so in these cases it is best to quickly identify or label the inappropriate behavior and then move on to the next task

Potential Assessment Measures for Levels V and VI

- Ross Information Processing Assessment
- Neurobehavioral Rating Scale
- Galveston Orientation and Amnesia Test
- Disability Rating Scale
- Functional Independence Measure and Functional Assessment Measure
- Portland Adaptability Inventory
- Rudimentary cognitive and neuropsychological screening with particular emphasis on insight/Awareness, Attention and Concentration, Impulsivity and distractibility, short-term Memory, and basic reasoning and organizational skills

- AUTOMATIC-APPROPRIATE (Level VII): Patient appears appropriate and oriented; is able to complete daily routine; shows increased Awareness of self and others but insight is superficial; patient overestimates abilities; judgment and Problem Solving are decreased; patient does not deal well with transitions or when routine is disrupted; irritability and Personality changes may be evident; Memory and rapid information processing are decreased; emphasis on home and community management may be appropriate

- PURPOSEFUL-APPROPRIATE (Level VIII): Patient exhibits carry-over of new learning and is able to integrate past and recent events in his or her current situation; relative to the patient's premorbid state, Memory, Problem Solving, judgment, and tolerance for stress may be decreased; psychosocial dysfunction, particularly within the family, may be noted; insight and Awareness may still be less than optimal; Personality changes may be apparent to those who knew the patient premorbidly; Depression may increase for the patient and family members; Vocational Rehabilitation activities may be appropriate

Treatment Suggestions for Levels VII and VIII

- Goals for these Rancho Levels are to increase the patient's ability to respond to minimal structure, to increase Awareness of cognitive and behavioral functioning (and to use compensatory strategies as appropriate), to increase psychosocial adaptation, and to integrate the individual into functional activities within the home, community, and work environment, if possible
- Emphasize functional living skills, community reintegration, and Vocational Rehabilitation
- Encourage use of compensatory Memory strategies and orthotics
- Monitor psychosocial and behavioral functioning (particularly anger control and self-centeredness); provide Behavior Management or Social Skills Training as appropriate for behavioral maladjustment
- Determine the patient's specific cognitive strengths and weaknesses and continue with formal Cognitive Rehabilitation as needed
- Give patient concrete and specific feedback about current problems and progress
- Patients must be included in the process of treatment planning and agree with the goals of rehabilitation
- Relate treatment goals and objectives to how they will improve the patient's quality of life (at these stages

patients must see that the goals and treatment in rehabilitation are relevant to their daily lives)

- Monitor the family's Adjustment and coping strategies (it is often in the second half of the first posttraumatic year that family distress heightens as family members realize that some cognitive and Personality changes in their loved one may be enduring)
- Encourage families and patients to make use of support groups offered by local chapters of the National Brain Injury Association
- Encourage patients and families to adopt a daily routine to keep their lives as predictable as possible (see Family Funtioning entry)
- Refer patients for Vocational Rehabilitation if appropriate
- Refer patients to Social Security for possible disability benefits if an extended period of disability is anticipated
- Monitor and treat as necessary psychological problems such as Depression and Anxiety in both the patient and the family (referral to a mental health professional may be necessary)
- Help patients structure their leisure or free time as this a frequent problem postinjury
- If a problem premorbidly, monitor and treat substance/alcohol use (see Alcohol Effects)
- Monitor patients' Motivation for and compliance with treatment; these issues are crucial for rehabilitation to be effective and become very important during this stage of recovery
- Encourage patients, if appropriate, to volunteer their time in nonstressful settings or to return to work part-time or at a lower level to test skills
- For children and adolescents, school and social reintegration will be critical (see Traumatic Brain Injury-Pediatric and School Placement/Considerations)
- Help patients find ways to be productive and feel good about themselves

- Do not give up hope or suggest that patients will never improve
- For problems with initation and drive, see Abulia, Executive Functions, Motivation, and Frontal Lobes

Potential assessment measures for Levels VII and VIII

- Portland Adaptability Inventory
- Neurobehavioral Rating Scale
- Disability Rating Scale
- Functional Independence Measure and Functional Assessment Measure
- The full range of cognitive and neuropsychological assessment instruments with emphasis on higher level skills and prediction of home/vocational functioning

Hagen, C., & Malkmus, D. (1979). *Intervention strategies for language disorders secondary to head trauma.* Atlanta: American Speech-Language-Hearing Association.

Reading. See Alexia, Dyslexia.

Reduplicative Paramnesia. A fixed Delusion in which patients believe that the place they are in has been duplicated; patients usually recognize and remember the name of the hospital or institution they are in but they insist it is located in a different community or area, usually closer to their home; patients cannot be globally amnestic to be diagnosed with this disorder and are often oriented in other spheres; pathology in the Frontal Lobe or the Right Hemisphere most often accompanies this disorder.

Reticular Activating System (RAS). The RAS is a network of nerve fibers and cell bodies that controls wakefulness and sleep, level of alertness, Consciousness, and some muscle activity and postural tone; it is located in the Brain Stem; damage to the RAS may result in Coma and decreased levels of Arousal.

Retrograde Amnesia. A loss of Memory (Amnesia) for events that occurred before the brain injury or the neurologic disorder; this type of Amnesia in TBI may be a few seconds (or nonexistent) or may extend for weeks to months; it is always shorter than Posttraumatic Amnesia (PTA) and is generally not a good predictor of outcome; during recovery, retrograde Amnesia may "shrink" so that events closer to the time of the injury are recalled better; following resolution of PTA, if retrograde Amnesia is longer than PTA and extends to the patient's childhood then a psychological cause is likely.

Rey Auditory Verbal Learning Test (RAVLT). A list learning and rote memorization task in which a 15-item list is read five times to the patient followed by a distractor list and then the patient is asked for immediate and 20 to 30 minute delayed recall of the original words; it is a common neuropsychological measure of Memory and learning used with persons with TBI; a similar task is the California Verbal Learning Test.

Lezak, M. D. (1995). *Neuropsychological assessment* (3rd ed.). New York: Oxford University Press.

Rey Osterrieth Complex Figure. A complex geometric figure that the patient is asked to copy (in some administrations patients are also asked to draw the design from Memory immediately after copying it and then again 30 minutes later); it is a measure of Constructional Abilities.

Lezak, M. D. (1995). *Neuropsychological assessment* (3rd ed.). New York: Oxford University Press.

Right Hemisphere Functioning. The right or nondominant hemisphere is critical for a number of abilities which individually or collectively can affect social behaviors, safety/judgment, and Perceptual Functioning; severe right hemisphere damage tends to result in more severe functional limitations than does damage to the left hemisphere where speech and language are dominant; a highly integrated and consistent approach to the rehabilitation of these patients is necessary; see also Lateralized Signs.

Potential Effects of Right Hemisphere Damage

- Left visual Neglect and spatial inattention

- Impaired Attention and Concentration
- Impulsivity
- Distractibility
- Impaired Awareness and insight into deficits and problems (Anosognosia) which can cause significant safety concerns (e.g., patients with left Neglect may think they are capable of driving or getting out of their wheelchair without help even though they are hemiplegic)
- Inability to appreciate the "big picture" or the gestalt of a situation or problem (these patients may perseverate on irrelevant detail or be unable to appreciate the impact of their injury on themselves and others)
- Impaired Perceptual Functioning
- Inability to appreciate nonverbal communication such as body posture or facial expressions
- Inability to appreciate the emotional tone in another's voice (Aprosodia) which may limit patients' ability to identify humor, anger, sarcasm, etc.
- Impaired Memory for nonverbal or visual information
- Spatial disorientation
- Inability to sequence activities or events
- Concrete Thinking
- Social insensitivity
- Inability to appreciate music
- Spatial Acalculia
- Flat Affect and an indifferent reaction to the environment
- A higher probablity of developing Hallucinations, Delusions, and Psychotic disorders than patients with left hemisphere lesions

Right Hemisphere Learning Disability. A constellation of nonverbal, visual, and often social learning problems that are developmental in origin and that may affect a child's academic and social functioning.

Rivermead Behavioral Memory Test. A Memory test designed to assess practical and behavioral aspects of Memory such as remembering names, faces, appointments, newspaper stories, a new route, and hidden belongings; it may be insensitive to subtle or higher level Memory disorders.

Wilson, B. A. (1986). *Rehabilitation of Memory.* New York: Guilford.

Ross Information Processing Assessment. A measure of cognitive linguistic deficits in adults and adolescents with TBI; it assesses basic communication and cognitive functions in 10 domains including Memory, Orientation, Problem Solving, organization, and auditory processing.

Ross, D. G. (1986). *Ross Information Processing Assessment Manual.* Austin, TX: Pro-Ed.

Scales of Cognitive Ability for Traumatic Brain Injury (SCATBI). A test battery designed to provide a systematic method of assessing cognitive deficits associated with TBI; there are five subtests that assess perception and discrimination, Orientation, organization, recall, and reasoning; the time to compete each subtest ranges from 10 minutes to 45 minutes.

Adamovich, B., & Hendersen, J. (1992). *Scales of Cognitive Ability for Traumatic Brain Injury Manual.* Chicago, IL: Riverside Publishing Company.

Schizophrenia. A major psychiatric illness that often results in significant disability for the patient; two or more of the following symptoms are characteristic of the disorder: Delusions, Hallucinations, disorganized speech, grossly disorganized or catatonic behavior, or "negative symptoms" such as paucity of speech, flat Affect, decreased initiation, etc.; onset is typically in late adolescence or early adulthood; persons with schizophrenia frequently have cognitive impairments.

School Placement/Considerations. Children who sustain TBI (see Traumatic Brain Injury-Pediatric) may have educational needs that require an IEP (Individualized Educational Program) in order to qualify for special education services, modified curricula, classroom modifications, etc.; schools are accustomed to providing services to children with Learning Disabilities or with Mental Retardation, both of which have different clinical presentations and course of symptoms than TBI (thus, school officials and even special educators are frequently unaware of the needs of children with TBI and how to meet their educational requirements).

Relevant Issues to Consider in School Re-entry for Children with TBI

- Decreased Attention and Concentration may affect a child's ability to remain focused in the classroom
- Impaired short-term Memory will have significant ramifications for new learning

- Children with TBI often exhibit decreased motor speed and coordination which can affect efficient note taking
- TBI in children can create "splintered skills" such that some abilities remain intact while others can be impaired
- Some previously learned abilities, such as reading comprehension or knowledge of math facts, can be unaffected by TBI, which can lead to some confusion for school officials who may then assume that all areas of the child's functioning are intact (the learning of new skills, however, may have been compromised)
- Achievement Tests and even Intelligence Tests are less sensitive to the effects of TBI than are neuropsychological measures of cognitive functioning
- Personality changes associated with TBI can alter a child's compliance with school and home rules as well as relationships with peers
- Depending on the age of the child at the time of injury, some skills may not have yet emerged which can result in impaired functioning in the future when these skills are taught
- Problems with organization can result from TBI which can interfere with completing homework on time, studying for tests, etc.
- Psychological and educational evaluations conducted by most school systems focus on IQ and Achievement Tests (abilities that may not be as vulnerable to TBI as other cognitive skills) and may not include measures of learning, Memory, mental processing speed, etc.
- Most children, even with severe brain injuries, "remember" their premorbid level of functioning and can be very sensitive to the type of academic support they receive and the type of classroom setting they are placed in
- Middle and high school students do not like to be identified as being different or having special needs which can make it very difficult to engage them in treatment or to give them special services

- Recovery from TBI is not a static process; children with TBI improve and so the IEP and services provided by the school also need to be flexible
- Rehabilitation professionals working with the child can only make recommendations or suggestions about educational planning, which the school is not required to follow; the parents must be the strongest and most vocal advocates for the child within the school system

Suggested Interventions to Assist Children with TBI with School Re-entry

- A major goal of school re-entry is to help the student avoid academic and social failure during the recovery time while not fostering overdependence on accommodations
- Begin communicating with school officials as soon as possible, even if return to school is unlikely in the immediate future
- Invite appropriate school personnel to begin tutoring the child, if clinically appropriate, even if the child is still in the hospital (this will allow for informal assessment and review of the child's fund of previously learned information)
- A comprehensive neuropsychological evaluation is suggested to clearly define the child's strengths and weaknesses and to provide concrete suggestions to the school
- Specific learning and Memory strategies may need to be used to help the student absorb new information presented in the classroom
- If possible, integrate occupational, physical, and speech therapy services into the child's IEP within the school rather than pulling the student out of school for traditional outpatient services
- Establish a "contact person" with the school who will serve as the liaison between the school and the treatment team; this person must agree to disseminate all relevant information from the therapists and parents to the child's teachers, and from the teachers back to the parents and therapists

- Teachers must understand the necessity to report any problems to the school contact person who can convey the information to the therapists and parents
- Educate school personnel as appropriate about the effects of TBI, their relevance to academic performance, and the recovery process
- Emphasize that re-entry to school is not a one-time event in the child's life but that returning to school is a series of transitions that requires flexibility and accommodation to the child's changing needs
- Try to return the child back to school as soon as possible even if only on a part-time basis or for selected subjects that he or she will likely be more successful in
- Try to keep the child out of self-contained special education or behavior disorder classes (the student may begin to mimic inappropriate behaviors, and the effects on Motivation and self-concept are frequently very negative)
- Educate and counsel the child's peers and classmates, if appropriate, about the sequelae to TBI and how to respond to the student's inappropriate behaviors or comments
- Suggest environmental changes as necessary
  - Sit near the front
  - Reduce assignments
  - Choose courses that highlight the child's strengths
  - Allow for increased time to complete assignments or finish tests
  - Provide rest periods during the day
  - Tape record lectures
  - Borrow notes from classmates
  - Verbally administer exams and tests or use other testing formats such as true/false, matching, or multiple choice questions for the child who exhibits problems with Memory retrieval
- Provide an assignment book to the student to keep track of homework and upcoming exams which can be reviewed by a teacher at the end of the school day and by a parent at night (a teacher can also check in with the stu-

dent at the beginning of the day to ensure that he or she has all the necessary books and assignments for the day's classes)

- Remove academic supports and accommodations as the child recovers and give more responsibility to him or her as appropriate
- Maintain expectations for age-appropriate behavior in school
- Remember that it is easier to reduce academic help if the child no longer needs it than it is to get extra help if needed after the child returns to school
- Modify and update the child's IEP as necessary
- With the most severe brain injuries, a change in emphasis from purely academic pursuits to vocational and independent community skills may be necessary

Savage, R. C., Russo, D. C., & Gardner, R. (1997). Traumatic brain injury in children: Neuropsychological, behavioral, and educational issues. In J. Leon-Carrion (Ed.), *Neuropsychological rehabilitation: Fundamentals, innovations, and directions* (pp. 499–512). Delray Beach, FL: GR/St. Lucie Press.

Seizure(s). Uncontrolled electrochemical activity in the brain that may result in altered motor and/or sensory functioning and which can affect Arousal and Consciousness; also known as epilepsy.

- The risk of developing seizures following Traumatic Brain Injury varies from about 5% to 35% (the latter percentage reflects the higher rate for penetrating or open head injuries)
- If posttraumatic seizures do occur, then most (70–75%) develop within the first year with a decreased risk over the next 10 years
- Seizures may also develop following Cerebrovascular Accidents (there is a higher incidence of seizures with hemorrhagic than obstructive strokes), brain Tumors, Dementia, and brain infections such as Meningitis and Herpes Simplex Encephalitis

- Drug use and alcohol withdrawal may also be a cause of seizures
- Patients with TBI may be placed on Anticonvulsants for 6 months to 2 years as a preventative or prophylactic measure against developing seizures; the most commonly used medications are Phenytoin (Dilantin), Phenobarbitol, and Carbamazepine (Tegretol)
- Seizures may also develop in persons without any known cerebral trauma or without any obvious cause; this is known as ideopathic epilepsy
- The most common and effective treatment for seizures is medication; in a small minority of patients with intractible focal seizures, brain surgery may also be a treatment option
- Behavioral alterations may occur prior to a seizure, known as pre-ictal behavior, with the patient experiencing an aura (sensing odors, noises, Anxiety, etc. or a feeling that a seizure is about to occur); behavior following a seizure (post-ictal behavior) may be marked by confusion, lethargy, fatigue, Aphasia, Amnesia, or other changes in mental status and may last a few seconds to several hours
- For obvious reasons, seizures create significant distress for the patient and family due to the loss of control and the unpredictability of the event; however, if well controlled by medication, seizures should not interfere significantly with a patient's recovery or level of independence
- Posttraumatic seizures can be exacerbated by alcohol use, fatigue, sleep deprivation, excessive stress, dehydration, excessive caffeine use, or failure to take anticonvulsant medications (patients should be educated about these issues)
- In extreme cases, some patients with a Temporal Lobe focus to their seizures may develop distinctive Personality characteristics such as humorlessness, hypergraphia (excessive writing), hyperreligiosity, hyposexuality, and interpersonal viscosity or interpersonal "stickiness"

Seizure Classification

- *Partial seizures:* This seizure type is initially focal or localized and starts in a circumscribed portion of one brain hemisphere; partial seizures are the most common type of seizures associated with brain trauma; there are three basic types of partial seizures
  - *Simple partial seizures:* There is no altered Consciousness but there are motor (e.g., rhythmic jerking of a body part) and sensory (e.g., burning or tingling feelings; auditory, visual, or olfactory sensations) symptoms
  - *Complex partial seizures:* Also sometimes referred to as Temporal Lobe epilepsy, these seizures may begin with the motor and sensory symtoms of simple partial seizures but eventually alter Consciousness (patient may be dazed or inattentive) or Consciousness may be impaired from the onset; Automatisms may also occur with this seizure type
  - *Partial seizure evolving to secondary generalized seizures:* These seizures begin as simple partial or complex partial seizures but spread through the Corpus Callosum and generalize to both hemispheres
- *Generalized seizures:* Seizures in which both hemispheres are involved; if such involvement occurs from the onset of the seizure then it is referred to as primarily generalized and if it occurs after a partial seizure, then it is referred to as secondarily generalized
  - *Convulsive or tonic-clonic seizures:* These seizures are known generally as grand mal and are characterized by an immediate loss of Consciousness and a marked increase in muscle tone or by repetitive jerks of the extremities and/or trunk; there are several variations of this type of seizure
  - *Nonconvulsive or absence seizures:* Known as petit mal seizures, these seizures are characterized by a sudden but relatively brief interruption of ongoing activities, usually with a staring spell; these are most common in

children between the ages of 4 and 12 and seldom persist into adulthood

Bennett, T. L. (Ed.). (1992). *The neuropsychology of epilepsy*. New York: Plenum Press.

Monaco, F. (1997). Posttraumatic seizures and post-traumatic epilepsy: Pharmacological prophylaxis and treatment. In J. Leon-Carrion (Ed.), *Neuropsychological rehabilitation: Fundamentals, innovations, and directions* (pp. 253–262). Delray Beach, FL: GR/St. Lucie Press.

Sensory Strip. The first Gyrus in the Parietal Lobes and just Posterior to the Central Sulcus; it receives sensory/tactile information from the contralateral side of the body; it is also known as the postcentral gyrus; see Cerebrum.

Shunt. A tube usually placed in one of the lateral Ventricles to drain excess Cerebrospinal Fluid from the brain to another body cavity, such as the peritoneal, due to Hydrocephalus; the shunt name commonly includes where it originates and where it ends (e.g., VP shunt for ventriculoperitoneal shunt).

Similarities. A subtest on the Wechsler Adult Intelligence Scale—Revised and the Wechsler Intelligence Scale for Children—III that assesses Abstract and Conceptual Thinking by asking the person to explain what each pair of words has in common (e.g., "arm-leg"); it is a good measure of general mental abilities and is sensitive to diffuse brain damage including Dementia and severe TBI; it is also affected by educational level.

Single Photon Emission Computed Tomography (SPECT). A functional neuroimaging procedure that measures regional cerebral blood flow and metabolic activity; this procedure is very similar to the Positron Emission Tomography (PET scan) although SPECT uses more readily available radioisotopes that do not require a special apparatus to prepare; as a result SPECT is much less expensive and more available for clinical use (the resolution of the anatomic images, however, is superior with PET than with SPECT).

Sleep Disorder. An alteration in the usual pattern of sleep that may be due to psychological/emotional causes such as Depression or Anxiety, medical factors such as pain or drug use, or neurologic conditions such as TBI, Dementia, or Cerebrovascular Accidents.

- Normal sleep architecture is divided into two distinct phases: rapid eye movement sleep and nonrapid eye movement sleep
  - *Rapid eye movement sleep* (REM) is synonymous with dreaming and increased autonomic nervous system activity; eye movements are rapid although the rest of the body is flaccid; EEG recordings are similar to wakefulness; the first REM sleep period usually begins about 90 to 120 minutes after the individual falls asleep (known as REM latency) and may last only about 10 minutes followed by nonrapid eye movement sleep; REM periods occur four to five times nightly and are progressively longer and more frequent
  - *Nonrapid eye movement sleep* (NREM) is divided into four stages that are distinguished by progressively greater depths of unconsciousness (slower, higher-voltage EEG patterns, such as delta waves, occur with deeper stages of NREM sleep); the eyes have slow rolling motions and muscle tone is present; deep NREM sleep provides most of the physical recuperative benefits of sleep; after passing through the four stages of NREM, the person returns to REM sleep followed again by NREM (this NREM-REM cycle repeats itself throughout the night in about 90 minute intervals)
- Adults average about 6 to 8 hours of total sleep time per night with about 20–28% in REM sleep
- With age, people tend to spend less time sleeping and less time in REM sleep; in the elderly, nighttime sleep is shorter and fragmented by multiple brief awakenings (see Age Effects)
- Sleep is controlled most by structures in the Brain Stem, Hypothalamus, and Thalamus

- Identifying sleep disorders is important because they can affect a patient's cognition (Attention, Mental Speed, Memory), psychological functioning (Depression, irritability, etc.), and ability to participate in therapy due to fatigue and sleepiness

Most Common Types of Sleep Disorders

- *Initial insomnia:* inability to fall asleep
- *Impaired sleep maintenance:* inability to remain asleep after falling asleep or being unable to fall back to sleep after awakening
- *Early morning awakening:* waking up early in the morning without being able to return to sleep (often present with Depression)
- *Excessive daytime sleepiness:* excessive fatigue and sleepiness during the day
- *Sleep apnea:* one of the most common causes of excessive daytime sleepiness, it is characterized by multiple, 10-second to 2-minute interruptions in breathing during sleep that results in partial awakenings although the person is unaware of these events (sleep apnea has been associated with impaired Attention and Concentration)
- *Narcolepsy:* brief, irresistible sleep episodes or attacks that can occur daily during routine activities

Sleep Problems and Neurologic Disorders

- Traumatic Brain Injury
  - With damage occurring at the level of the Brain Stem, sleep architecture can be affected, including decreased REM sleep, alpha wave intrusions, and disruption of sleep stages
  - The most frequent subjective sleep problem for TBI patients with ongoing cognitive complaints is poor sleep maintenance
  - Excessive daytime sleepiness is most common during the acute stages of recovery from TBI
  - Sleep apnea has been reported following TBI
  - The presence of pain (headaches, neck pain, etc.) increases the number of sleep complaints twofold

- Dementia
  - In the middle to late stages, Dementia can disrupt or invert sleep-wake cycles and produce nighttime confusion, disorientation, and Agitation (known as the sundown syndrome)
  - Sleep latency can also be lengthened which decreases sleep efficiency
- Cerebrovascular Accidents
  - An inversion of the sleep-wake cycle can occur, particularly during the acute recovery phase
  - Sleep apnea and changes with sleep architecture have also been reported with this population
- Multiple Sclerosis
  - Persons with MS tend to have complaints of initial insomnia and problems with sleep maintenance which may be due to both neurologic factors and Depression
- Many other conditions such as Depression, Schizophrenia, alcoholism, Seizures, Mania, and medication side effects can also contribute to sleep problems

Assessment and Behavioral Treatment of Sleep Problems

- If an inpatient, monitor the patient's sleep during the night at 15- or 30-minute intervals (also observe for apnea episodes) and also during the day (monitor for 3 days with formal "sleep charting")
- Determine the patient's premorbid sleep history and try to conform the patient's daily schedule within the hospital to his or her routine at home (e.g., time to get up in the morning, nap schedule)
- Rule out medical or medication effects that could be affecting sleep patterns
- Rule out psychological or emotional problems that could be contributing to poor sleep
- In patients with intractible sleep problems, consider referral for polysomnography (sleep study)
- Try to control the stimuli associated with sleep by avoiding naps during the day (if the patient is not sleeping at

night), using the bed only for sleep and not while reading, watching TV, or socializing, going to bed only when sleepy, keeping bright lights on at times of sleepiness during the day, maintaining a schedule for time spent in bed and adhering to it even on weekends, and keeping noise and lights low while trying to sleep

Beetar, J. T., Guilmette, T. J., & Sparadeo, F. R. (1996). Sleep and pain complaints in symtomatic traumatic brain injury and neurologic populations. *Archives of Physical Medicine and Rehabilitation, 77*, 1298–1302.

Espinar-Sierra, J. (1997). Treatment and rehabilitation of sleep disorders in patients with brain damage. In J. Leon-Carrion (Ed.), *Neuropsychological rehabilitation: Fundamentals, innovations, and directions* (pp. 263–281). Delray Beach, FL: GR/St. Lucie Press.

Kaufman, D. M. (1995). *Clinical neurology for psychiatrists.* Philadelphia, PA: W. B. Saunders Company.

Social Skills Training. A behavioral intervention or program designed to improve social and interpersonal behaviors in persons with TBI whose abilities in this area have been diminished by their injury; problems with Agitation, Aggression, self-centeredness, passivity, etc. are not uncommon problems with TBI and require behavioral and psychosocial interventions to alter; deficient social skills can interfere significantly with the patient's ability to hold a job, maintain friendships, live with family members, obtain what he or she wants from others, and maintain self-esteem; social skills training can occur during the usual course of therapy or can be a more formal and distinct program; see also Behavior Management entry.

- Some specific goals for social skills training may include the patient's ability to:
  - Start, maintain, and finish a conversation
  - Follow instructions
  - Express him- or herself negatively when appropriate to do so
  - Accept criticism or consequences of one's actions
  - Withstand interruptions

- Express and receive appreciation, love, praise, and affection
- Receive fair treatment as a consumer
- Disagree appropriately
- Ask others for favors
- Defend one's own rights

General Principles in Social Skills Training

- The training should be included as part of a more global rehabilitation program
- Retraining social skills can be a formal, distinct program with specific trainers *or* it can be carried out during the course of routine treatment (e.g., occupational, physical, speech, and recreational therapy sessions) by clinicians who usually work with the patient
- The "trainers" should think of themselves as teachers or coaches
- Social skills can be learned and practiced
- The use of social skills is based on the individual's ability to choose freely his or her course of action but being able to recognize the consequences of one's actions
- It is important for family and friends to reinforce, practice, and give feedback to patients regarding their interpersonal behavior
- The training needs to consider the person's cognitive strengths and weaknesses (work with the patient's strengths)
- Positive praise and social reinforcement can be powerful in altering behavior
- Improving patients' insight and Awareness about their interpersonal behavior is a crucial step in improving social skills
- A minimal level of cognitive ability is necessary for formal social skills training to be effective (e.g., patients need to be out of Posttraumatic Amnesia, able to attend to instruction for 15 or more minutes, learn and recall some new information)

- Priority should be given to those skills that are most necessary to be able to give and receive social support

Social Skills Training During the Course of Routine Treatment

- The team should agree on the specific behaviors to be targeted for intervention
  - Choose behaviors (not attitudes unless they can be defined in behavioral terms) that are concrete and observable to all
  - Be modest—begin with only one or two goals
  - Consider the patient's premorbid social functioning and do not target behaviors that are incompatible with the patient's history
- Try to ignore all inappropriate behaviors that are not actively targeted unless they threaten the health of the patient or the health or property of others
- Inform the patient in a matter-of-fact fashion about the plan to target specific behaviors and why
- Help patients understand the connection between their injury and their maladaptive behaviors, the consequences of their behavior (e.g., offends others, isolates patient), the understanding that it is difficult for them to control or modify these actions (e.g., don't "blame" patients for their "bad" behavior), and why you think this type of intervention will help
- Use verbal praise for any behaviors that approximate change or show any effort on the patient's part to improve his or her social skills
- When the target behavior is exhibited, a structured interaction can be used to teach and then practice the social skill to replace the inappropriate behavior (the team should decide whether some or all of the following steps should be used, based on the cognitive functioning of the patient, the circumstances under which the behavior is exhibited, and the degree to which the patient's behavior interferes with his or her social functioning); some or all of the following steps can be used

- Use the patient's name in the sentence
- Speak to the patient in a matter-of-fact matter and do not show anger, disgust, or embarrassment
- State specifically the maladaptive behavior exhibited
- Explain the consequences of the behavior
- State specifically the correct thing to do
- Explain the desirable consequences of using the correct behavior
- Determine if the patient understands the information
- Practice the new behavior (if possible at that time)
- Verbally praise and reinforce the patient for the correct behavior

- Inform the family of the interventions and enlist their support in changing the target behavior

Social Skills Training as a Distinct and Separate Program

- Evaluate the patient's neuropsychological status
- Assess the patient's social competence
    - Determine the strengths and weaknesses of the patient's method of social interaction
    - Discuss with family and friends their impressions and concerns about the patient's social behavior
    - Assess how the patient evaluates his or her own social functioning
    - Determine the patient's premorbid social functioning
- Establish individual behavioral goals that are compatible with the patient's history and that interfere with the patient's social needs
- Treat social skills in groups or classes rather than in individual sessions
- Begin addressing behaviors that are least disruptive and easiest to change
- Formally instruct patients about proper social behavior, emphasizing the patient's individual goals, including the appropriate use of body posture, tone of voice, word usage, etc.

- Discuss the benefits of appropriate social behavior for each specific instruction
- Model the correct behavior for the patient and discuss how the behavior of the model could be altered to improve or worsen the social interaction
- Have the patient role-play social behaviors while receiving specific instructions from the trainer
- Have the patient practice social behaviors without overt instruction from the trainer but provide him or her ample and concrete feedback about the interaction
- Emphasize and discuss the patient's own Awareness of his or her social skills and their effect on others
- Ask patients to monitor and record their social interactions outside of the formal training sessions
- Reward and reinforce patients when they have used trained behaviors in real life situations

Blackerby, W. F., & Gualtieri, T. (1991). Recent advances in neurobehavioral rehabilitation. *NeuroRehabilitation, 1,* 53–61.

Machuca, R., Carrasco, M., Gonzalez, A. M., Rodriguez-Duarte, R., & Leon-Carrion, J. (1997). Training for social skills after brain injury. In J. Leon-Carrion (Ed.), *Neuropsychological rehabilitation: Fundamentals, innovations, and directions* (pp. 453–468). Delray Beach, FL: GR/St. Lucie Press.

Spinal Accessory Nerve. Cranial Nerve XI; one of a group of Bulbar Nerves that originates in the Medulla, the Spinal Accessory Nerve controls the sternocleidomastoid muscles and the upper portion of the trapezius muscles which allows for movement of the chin and shoulders.

Stereognosis. The ability to recognize objects by touch; see Astereognosis.

Stimulus Bound. The inability to screen out irrelevant stimuli; to be "pulled" or respond to a stimulus regardless of its relevancy in solving a problem; reflects an inability to shift Attention and regulate behavior; usually associated with Frontal Lobe or Executive Function deficits.

Striatum. One of the components of the Basal Ganglia.

Stroke. Another name for Cerebrovascular Accident (CVA).

Stroop Color-Word Test. A test in which patients are asked to name the color of ink a different color word is printed in (e.g., the word "red" is printed in green ink and the patient is asked to name the color [green] and not the word [red]); it is designed to assess Concentration and the ability to inhibit the more automatic response of reading the word rather than naming the color; there are different versions of the Stroop available; it can be sensitive to neurologic disorders including TBI.

Stupor. See Arousal.

Subarachnoid. The space below the Arachnoid Layer but above the Pia Mater that contains Cerebrospinal Fluid; bleeding into the subarachnoid space is referred to as a Subarachnoid Hemorrhage; blood in the subarachnoid space typically results in acute neurologic symptoms and can be fatal; see Subdural and Subdural Hemorrhage.

Subarachnoid Hemorrhage (SAH). A Hemorrhage or bleeding in the Subarachnoid space (i.e., below the Arachnoid Layer) due most commonly to ruptured Aneurysms; initial symptoms frequently include severe headache, nausea, vomiting, and neck stiffness; blood in the Subarachnoid space, which may travel over and between the brain convexities, is an irritant to brain tissue; SAH can be life-threatening and may result in long-term cognitive deficits.

Subcortical Structures. Structures that lie beneath the cerebral Cortex such as the Basal Ganglia, Thalamus, Hippocampus, and Amygdala; lesions to these structures may result in impaired motor functioning as well as decreased Mental Speed, impaired Memory, and slowed reaction time; Parkinson's and Huntington's Diseases are examples of "subcortical dementias"; see Figure 8 for the location of some of these structures.

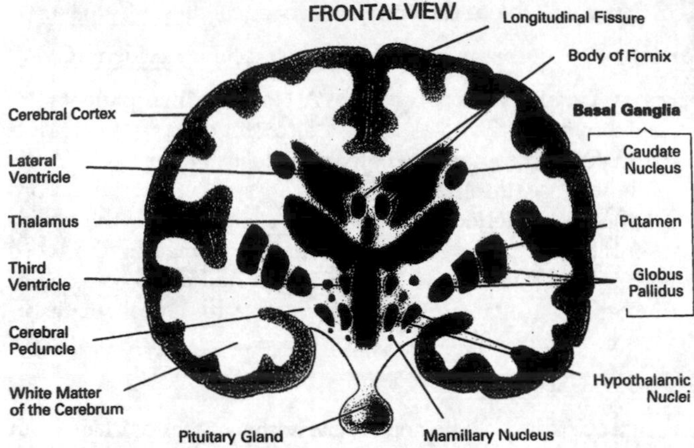

Figure 8. Cross section of the brain displaying several subcortical structures. (Reprinted with permission from Neurological Reference Guide. [Promotional cards]. Warner-Lambert Company, Morris Plains, NJ.)

Subdural. The space below the Dura but above the Arachnoid Layer; bleeding into this space is referred to as a Subdural Hematoma or Hemorrhage.

Subdural Hematoma (SDH). A collection of blood in the Subdural space (i.e., below the Dura but above the Arachnoid Layer) caused most frequently by head trauma; because the blood is venous in origin, it tends to collect more slowly than Subarachnoid or Epidural Hematomas which develop from arterial blood supplies (due to brain Atrophy in the elderly, a SDH after head injury may take several weeks to develop because the cranial vault is able to accommodate the space that the Hematoma occupies); a SDH may need to be drained neurosurgically if it displaces or pushes other brain structures; because the blood accumulates above the Arachnoid layer, it does not come into direct contact with the Cortex of the brain and thus does not present with the same neurologic symptoms as a Subarachnoid Hemorrhage; (see Mass Effect and Midline Shift).

Sylvian Fissure. The large sulcus or groove that separates the Temporal Lobe from the Frontal Lobe.

Symbol Search. One of the subtests of the Wechsler Intelligence Scale for Children—III which assesses visual searching/scanning under timed conditions.

Temporal Lobes. The lobes located on the sides or lateral portions of the brain (see Cerebrum for diagram); both Temporal Lobes are associated with olfaction and odor perception; the Hippocampus (a brain structure necessary for short term Memory) is located within the inside fold of each Temporal Lobe, which makes this brain area very important in storing ongoing information and recent events; the Temporal Lobes also contain brain structures that are part of the Limbic System (see also Mammillary Bodies and Amygdala) which are further associated with Memory, emotional functioning, and drive states; see also Kluver-Bucey Syndrome.

- *Left temporal lobe functions*: auditory comprehension (see Aphasia); verbal Memory; word or information retrieval
- *Right temporal lobe functions*: nonverbal sound recognition and discrimination (see Agnosia); sequencing and organization; nonverbal or visual Memory; recognition and perception of tones and melody in music as well as tone of voice and inflection (see Aprosodia)

Temporal Lobe Epilepsy (TLE). Seizures that originate in the Temporal Lobes and which may result in altered Mood, Hallucinations, Automatisms, and Personality changes; see also complex partial Seizures.

Test Scores. The scale or method used to report performance on evaluations or assessments (in this case on tests of cognitive or neuropsychological, language, or perceptual functioning).

Common Test Terms

- *Mean*: an average or middle score obtained by adding all the scores together and dividing by the number of cases
- *Median*: another way of calculating an average or middle score; it is the score that falls in the middle when all test scores are ranked from lowest to highest
- *Mode*: the score that occurs most frequently
- *Standard deviation*: the degree to which a score deviates from the mean (either above it or below it); scores that fall within one standard deviation of the mean include 68%

of the group or sample that the test was normed on (34% fall above the mean and 34% fall below the mean); scores that fall within two standard deviations of the mean include 98% of the group or sample that the test was normed on; scores that fall within three standard deviations of the mean include greater than 99% of the sample or group

- *Raw score*: the person's actual performance on a specific test; it may be the number of items right or wrong, the amount of time to complete the test, etc.; it is a relatively meaningless number without knowing how it relates to the raw scores obtained by other people with or without neurologic dsyfunction
- *Normative group*: the group of subjects (usually normal, nonclinical samples) used to establish what a "normal" performance is on a specific test; may also be known as a standardization sample or population
- *Percentile rank*: a method of ranking an individual's score with other persons in the normative group (e.g., a score that falls at the 25th percentile is higher than 25% of the people on whom the test was normed; a score at the 87th percentile is higher than 87% of the normative sample, etc.)
- *Standard scores*: a method of reporting test scores for which the mean and standard deviation are known (and from which percentile ranks can be calculated); it allows for a common language to be used when reporting test performance; there are several different types of standard scores, some of which are:
  - T-scores: based on a mean of 50 and a standard deviation of 10
  - IQ scores: based on a mean of 100 and a standard deviation of 15
  - IQ subtest scores: based on a mean of 10 and a standard deviation of 3
  - z-scores: based on a mean of 0 and a standard deviation of 1
- Figure 9 graphically displays the distribution of different standard scores and their relationship to percentile ranks and standard deviations

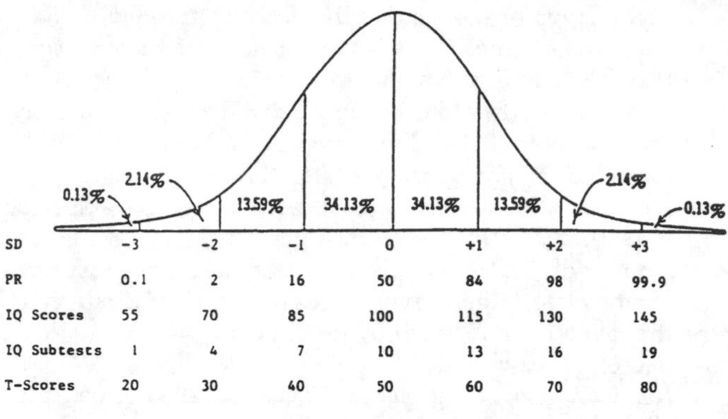

Figure 9. Distribution of commonly used test scores and percentile rankings in the normal curve. SD = standard deviation (SD = 0 is the mean). PR = Percentile ranking. IQ subsets = Wechsler IQ subtest standard scores. The percentages under the curve represent the percent of cases or scores found within each standard deviation (e.g., 34.13% of scores fall between the mean and + 1 standard deviation). (Reprinted with permission from *Traumatic Brain Injury: Evaluation and Litigation* by R. W. Petrocelli, T. J. Guilmette, and M. E. McNamara, 1994, p. 75. Copyright 1994 by The Michie Company. Charlottesville, VA: The Michie Co.)

Thalamus. Two Subcortical Structures that lie on each side of the third Ventricle and serve as a major relay station for sensory information to the Cortex; it has rich connections to the Frontal Lobes so damage to the Thalamus can affect many facets of neurobehavioral functioning.

- It is important for rudimentary functions such as Arousal but perhaps more important for responsiveness and Awareness to the environment

- The thalamus is also important for new learning (recent or short-term Memory) and also for recall of past information or long-term Memory with a temporal gradient (i.e., information that is learned more recently or closer in time to before the brain damage is less likely to be recalled than information learned earlier)
- Extensive bilateral thalamic damage can cause severe Anterograde Amnesia (such as seen in Korsakoff's Syndrome) as well as some Retrograde Amnesia
- Thalamic damage can also affect emotional and behavioral functioning with damage possibly resulting in Apathy or Abulia, decreased drive and spontaneity, or Impulsivity and Disinhibition
- Left sided thalamic damage may result in decreased language abilities (and perhaps verbal Memory problems) and right thalamic damage may produce some impairment with Perceptual Functioning, including left Neglect (and perhaps visual Memory problems)

Tinnitus. A noise in the ears such as ringing, whistling, buzzing, etc.; it can be caused by Tumors, Traumatic Brain Injury (usually more common in mild than severe TBI), Ischemia, and damage to the inner ear; the cochlear division of the Acoustic Nerve (Cranial Nerve VIII) would be implicated.

Token Economy. A complex Behavior Management system designed to increase appropriate behaviors through the use of operant conditioning or rewards.

- Patients are given tokens for exhibiting specific behaviors and these tokens can be "traded in" for other, more tangible rewards such as candy, television time, magazines, etc.
- It requires a high degree of control of the patient's environment, a staff highly trained in Behavior Management techniques, careful monitoring of the patient's behavior and consequences, and a lengthy period of time to work with the patient
- It likely is most effective with adolescents or with patients who will be in a controlled environment for an extended period of time

- The use of rewards/incentives can be applied to many behavioral problems without creating a formal token economy system (see Behavior Management)

Trail Making Test. A paper and pencil test sensitive to brain damage which is designed to assess Attention, Concentration, Mental Speed, and visual scanning; it is composed of Parts A and B (Part A requires the subject to connect in ascending order numbers scattered on a page and Part B requires the subject to alternately connect in ascending order numbers and letters scattered on a page).

Transient Ischemic Attack (TIA). A temporary disruption in Cerebral Circulation that can cause physical and cognitive impairments; TIAs can last from a few seconds to hours although symptoms must dissipate within 24 hours to be considered a TIA (if symptoms persist beyond 24 hours then it is considered a Cerebrovascular Accident); if left untreated, about 5% to 25% of individuals with a TIA will develop a CVA within 1 year.

Kaufman, D. M. (1995). *Clinical neurology for psychiatrists.* Philadelphia, PA: W. B. Saunders Company.

Transient Global Amnesia (TGA). A sudden and transient loss of Memory resulting in Anterograde and some Retrograde Amnesia (the Retrograde Amnesia is usually for recently acquired information, such as the events that occurred in the last several hours or days); there are no accompanying physical deficits; TGAs may last from 3 to 24 hours and have a recurrence rate of about 10%; they are not caused by head trauma and thus are not referred to as Posttraumatic Amnesia; they may be precipitated by exertion; TGAs are believed to be caused by Transient Ischemic Attacks of the Basilar Artery which disrupt circulation of the Posterior Cerebral Arteries affecting Temporal Lobe functioning (see Circle of Willis and Cerebral Circulation).

Kaufman, D. M. (1995). *Clinical neurology for psychiatrists.* Philadelphia, PA: W. B. Saunders Company.

Traumatic Brain Inury (TBI)—Adult. A physiological disruption of brain function due to external trauma (the trauma may be the result of an object striking the head, by the head striking an object such as a windshield, or by sudden deceleration such as severe whiplash).

- TBI is the second leading cause of neurologic disability in adults in the U.S. (the first is Cerebrovascular Accidents) although it is the leading cause of disability for young adults
- The most common ages for sustaining a TBI are between 15 and 40
- Estimates of TBI vary although approximately 600,000 to 1,000,000 new cases per year are reported (motor vehicle accidents are the most common cause)
- Males are twice as likely as females to sustain a TBI
- Alcohol is a common contributing factor to TBI (see Alcohol Effects)
- If the Dura is penetrated, then the injury is referred to as an open head injury; if the Dura is not penetrated, then it is referred to as a closed head injury
- Recovery of function and level of disability occur in stages and may vary somewhat from person to person (see Ranchos Los Amigos Cognitive Scale)
- The National Brain Injury Association, known formerly as the National Head Injury Foundation (1–800–444–NHIF), has excellent educational materials for families and survivors of TBI and can also provide information about local affiliates for support groups, clinicians with expertise in TBI, referral information, etc.

Neuropathology of TBI

- Diffuse Axonal Injury is the most common source of neurobehavioral and cognitive dysfunction and can result in multifocal and global brain damage
- Focal Contusions and Hemorrhages (particularly to the Frontal and Temporal Lobes) can also be a source of morbidity
- Contrecoup Injuries may produce focal trauma far from the site of the initial injury

- Secondary injuries can further complicate and impede recovery
  - Anoxia (inadequate oxygen due to ruptured airways, facial injuries, pulmonary injuries, respiratory arrest, etc.)
  - Hydrocephalus
  - Edema (swelling of brain tissues due to collections of intracellular fluids, blood, etc.)
  - Multiple trauma and multiple system injuries
  - Seizures
  - Intoxication at the time of injury (see Alcohol Effects)
- Penetrating head injuries (from gunshot or knife wounds) typically cause only focal damage to those brain areas struck and tend not to produce the global or widespread cognitive deficits seen with Diffuse Axonal Injury

Classification and Severity of TBI

- TBIs are generally classified as mild, moderate, and severe (see Mild Traumatic Brain Injury as a separate entry for more extensive information)
- Most TBIs are mild (approximately 75%); moderate TBIs comprise about 15% of all injuries sustained and severe TBIs make up about 10%
- The injury parameters for mild TBI are generally agreed upon although the distinctions between moderate and severe TBI are less clear
- Severity of TBI is based generally based upon admitting Glasgow Coma Scale (GCS), length of loss of consciousness (LOC or Coma), and length of Posttraumatic Amnesia (PTA)
- A method of classifying TBI severity is:

Variable	*Mild*	*Moderate*	*Severe*
Admitting GCS	13–15	9–12	3–8
LOC	< 30 min, if at all	30 min–6 hrs	>6 hrs
PTA	< 24 hrs	1–7 days	>7 days

- Neuroimaging results (e.g., CT scans and Magnetic Resonance Imaging) can also be used as a measure of injury severity although CT scans are the diagnostic procedure of choice because they can be obtained quickly and are readily available
  - It is important to remember that imaging studies, such as CT scans, measure brain *structures* and not brain *functions*
  - Patients with severe TBI and who are in Coma may have normal CT scans
  - CT scans can detect only gross structural changes and are poor at imaging lower brain structures, such as the Brain Stem

Predicting Outcome

- No single measure of injury severity (or even combinations of injury parameters) can provide a fully reliable estimate of long-term outcome from TBI
- Outcome can vary greatly from person to person as moderate to severe TBI does not necessarily produce a homogeneous group of residual impairments
- Outcome depends on several factors, in addition to the severity of the injury, including premorbid cognitive and Personality functioning, family and social supports, availability of rehabilitation, age at injury, etc.
- Although quicker rates of recovery are usually associated with better long-term outcomes, there is no specific "recovery window" beyond which further improvement will not occur (anecdotal evidence suggests that some improvement, albeit subtle, may continue for years)
- Damage to specific brain structures, such as the Frontal Lobes, may impair specific abilities that interfere with adaptive skills
- Studies have revealed the following relationships between injury severity and outcome:
  - Neurobehavioral outcome at one year postinjury was most predicted by postresuscitation GCS and pupil reactivity

- Lower GCS scores and longer periods of Coma are generally related to worse outcome
- Coma of 2 weeks or more is infrequently associated with full recovery
- In the majority of cases, Coma of greater than 4 weeks is associated with severe disability at 1 year postinjury
- Longer periods of PTA are associated with poorer recovery
- PTA longer than 7 days has been associated with Memory problems in about half of patients studied
- With PTA longer than 4 weeks, patients rarely achieve a good recovery

- Approximately 20%–40% of persons with moderate to severe TBI are able to return to work or school in some capacity, although greater cognitive and personality impairments are associated with poorer vocational outcome (see Vocational Rehabilitation)

Physical Impairments

- Physical problems are typically the least disruptive and disabling symptoms associated with TBI
- The most common physical impairments associated with TBI include headache, dizziness, Tinnitus, changes in bladder and bowel functioning, Dysphagia, Dysarthria, Ataxia, increased muscle tone, Diplopia, fatigue, muscle weakness, Visual Field Cuts

Cognitive Impairments

- Cognitive deficits are frequently associated with greater disability than are physical impairments but may not be as debilitating as emotional and behavioral problems (see next section)
- Cognitive impairments following TBI may vary greatly; they may be readily apparent in casual conversation with the survivor of TBI or they may be more subtle and detectable only with specific tasks or with formal neuropsychological testing
- Some cognitive skills tend to be more resistant to TBI than others, including single word reading, vocabulary, fund of

long-term information or knowledge, and performance on selected subtests of standardized Intelligence Tests

- Cognitive problems will vary depending on what stage of recovery the patient is in, which specific brain areas may have been affected, the patient's premorbid skills, etc.
- During PTA, patients exhibit global confusion, disorientation, and at times Agitation
- In the absence of focal brain injury (e.g., to temporal and/or parietal structures), most language and perceptual functions return to normal levels by about 1 year posttrauma
- Residual or long-term cognitive deficits from TBI vary but may include the following:
  - Decreased Mental Speed or rate of information processing
  - Poor Concentration and an inability to sustain or shift Attention (e.g., distractibility)
  - Short-term Memory deficits with particular problems absorbing and/or retrieving new information
  - Concrete Thinking and poor Problem Solving or judgment
  - Deficits with Executive Functioning

Emotional and Behavioral Impairments

- Personality changes are some of the most debilitating problems following TBI and frequently lead to significant family burden/distress as well as impaired social and vocational functioning
- Social isolation and lack of ability to structure free time are frequent complaints from persons with TBI and their families
- The major "active" behavioral disturbances following TBI have been summarized by Prigatano (1992) as including the following:
  - Irritability
  - Agitation
  - Belligerence
  - Anger
  - Abrupt and unexpected acts of violence or episodic dyscontrol

- Impatience
- Restlessness
- Inappropriate social responses
- Emotional Lability (see Affect)
- Sensitivity to noise or distress
- Anxiety
- Delusions
- Paranoia
- Mania or manic-like states

- The major "passive" behavioral disturbances following TBI have been summarized by Prigatano (1992) as including the following:
  - Aspontaneity
  - Sluggishness
  - Loss of interest in the environment
  - Loss of drive or initiative (see Abulia)
  - Fatigue
  - Depression
  - Childishness (self-centered behavior, insensitivity to others, etc.)
  - Helplessness (requires supervision or continued cueing to accomplish goals)
  - Lack of insight (see Awareness)

Treatment Considerations

- In establishing treatment plans and goals, clinicians must consider the following:
  - The premorbid cognitive and Personality functioning of the individual
  - The expected sequelae given the type and severity of the injury, any complicating secondary conditions such as Anoxia, and evidence for any focal brain trauma noted clinically or from neurodiagnostic procedures
  - The current stage in the patient's recovery
  - Family Functioning, support, expectations, etc.
  - Current cognitive/neuropsychological deficits, physical limitations, and behavioral/emotional disorders

- Family education is very important to optimize outcome and adjustment to injury
- Consistency in treatment is crucial
- It is important to assist patients to find ways to be productive, even if in small ways
- In the early stages of recovery, the following entries may be helpful in providing specific treatment recommendations:
  - Coma
  - Rancho Los Amigos Cognitive Scale
  - Agitation
  - Attention
  - Orientation
  - Posttraumatic Amnesia
  - Behavior Management
  - Disinhibition
  - Cognitive Rehabilitation
- In the middle to late stages of recovery, the following entries may be helpful in providing specific treatment recommendations:
  - Rancho Los Amigos Cognitive Scale
  - Awareness
  - Attention
  - Impulsivity
  - Behavior Management
  - Behavior Contracts
  - Motivation
  - Memory
  - Abstract and Conceptual Thinking
  - Problem Solving
  - Social Skills Training
  - Perceptual Functioning
  - Cognitive Rehabilitation
  - Executive Functions and Frontal Lobes
  - Alcohol Effects
  - Adjustment (to disability or deficits)
  - Abulia
  - Depression

- Anxiety
- Family Functioning
- Vocational Rehabilitation

Petrocelli, R. W., Guilmette, T. J., & McNamara, M. E. (1994). *Traumatic brain injury: Evaluation and litigation*. Charlottesville, VA: The Michie Company.

Prigatano, G. P. (1992). Personality disturbances associated with traumatic brain injury. *Journal of Consulting and Clinical Psychology, 60*, 360-368.

Traumatic Brain Injury (TBI)—Pediatric. A physiological disruption of brain function due to external trauma (the trauma may be the result of an object striking the head, by the head striking an object such as a windshield, or by sudden deceleration such as severe whiplash).

- TBI is the leading cause of death in children and is a major cause of disability
- Falls, bicycle accidents, and motor vehicle accidents are the primary causes
- Some data suggest that premorbid functioning (i.e., history of Learning Disabilities, Attention Deficit Hyperactivity Disorder, etc.) is related to the incidence of TBI in children

Neuropathology of TBI in Children

- Similar to adults, Diffuse Axonal Injury is the most common underlying neuropathological condition in TBI
- Unlike adults, children are less vulnerable to developing mass lesions (e.g., Hematomas)
- Children have a greater capacity for survival than adults
  - In adults with Glasgow Coma Scale scores less than 8 there is a 30% to 50% mortality rate
  - In children with Glasgow Coma Scale scores less than 8 there is a 9% mortality rate
- Children are less likely to lose consciousness than adults
- Retrograde and Anterograde Amnesia are less common in children, particularly if under age 9

Issues Unique to Children

- Children are not simply smaller versions of adults; their cognitive, Personality, and psychosocial developments need to be considered in assessment and treatment

- Unlike in adults, the effects of the TBI on brain function interact with the maturation or development of the child
  - Skills that are emerging or developing may be affected differently by TBI than skills that are already established
  - Due to the multistaged and prolonged process of Frontal Lobe development, injury to these brain structures at an early age may result in delayed onset of impairments, particularly with interpersonal relationships, social behaviors, and vocational skills
  - Language deficits (Aphasia) may recover better if sustained at a younger age (e.g., less than 6 years of age) although a severe Memory deficit sustained at the same age would be devastating to the cognitive development of the child
- Family Functioning, particularly parental relationships, can affect outcome and treatment needs
- Assessment of cognitive/neuropsychological functioning must be accomplished with test instruments and procedures that are age-appropriate and normed on children and adolescents (do not use adult measures and try to extrapolate how the child performed)
- Psychosocial development such as peer relationships, the need for independence/dependence, etc. need to be considered in treating children and adolescents
- Returning to school where new learning is expected to occur may place increased demands on the child
- Adolescents who often have strong developmental needs to conform to their classmates or "fit in," routinely reject treatment because it sets them apart from their peers

Cognitive Impairments in Moderate to Severe TBI

- Effects on IQ and Intelligence Tests
  - There is usually a significant relationship between injury severity and IQ deficit
  - IQ seems more adversely affected when injury occurs at a younger age
  - IQ deficits and Coma duration seem most related for children less than 8 years old
  - Improvement in IQ has been noted for up to 5 years postinjury

  - IQ may decline significantly following severe TBI and may become somewhat "fixed" at the level obtained at the time of injury
  - Normal or average IQ does *not* rule out brain injury or damage (for example, IQ tests do not measure short-term Memory, a common cognitive impairment with TBI)
- Attention and Memory
  - Deficits in these areas occur with high frequency and have significant educational consequences
  - Speed of information processing or Mental Speed are very vulnerable to TBI
  - Short-term Memory impairments are common
- Language
  - Aphasia is infrequent
  - Linguistic disturbances are varied
  - Specific deficits are related to the degree to which specific skills have already been acquired
- Visual-motor speed and coordination are frequently reduced, which can have significant implications for note taking, finishing tests on time, etc.
- Problem Solving and organization
  - Problems in this area occur with variable frequency
  - May affect time management, organization with classroom assignments, etc.
  - Difficult to assess formally
- Academic areas such as reading, math, spelling, and written expression may be affected to varying degrees and will need to be evaluated and followed as necessary

Behavioral and Emotional Impairments in Moderate to Severe TBI

- A weak relationship, at most, with cognitive deficits
- Greater behavioral problems are associated with longer lengths of Coma
- The occurrence of TBI in children with behavior disorders is three times more likely than in normal controls
- There is no concensus about the most common types of deficits although the following have been reported:

- Aggressiveness and irritability
- Hyperactivity, restlessness, Impulsivity
- Social disinhibition
- Emotional volatility
- Social withdrawal and isolation
- Altered self-concept and self-esteem (Depression)

Treatment Suggestions for Moderate to Severe TBI

- During acute recovery, behavioral and environmental management of Agitation, confusion, and disorientation will be necessary (see also Orientation, Posttraumatic Amnesia (PTA), and Children's Orientation and Amnesia Test)
- Children become especially fearful in unfamiliar environments, such as hospitals, so try to make their room as "friendly" as possible with familiar pictures, favorite posters, stuffed animals, games, etc.
- Encourage family and parental involvement (during hospitalization a parent may need to stay with younger children on a 24-hour basis)
- Educate family members about TBI and support them emotionally, including the child's siblings who will tend to feel excluded or "left out"
- When PTA clears for a school-aged child, begin reviewing academic work and skills that were already mastered prior to the injury
- A comprehensive neuropsychological assessment will be necessary to identify the child's cognitive strengths and weaknesses
- Cognitive Rehabilitation activities must be age-appropriate and of interest to the child (younger children will not tolerate drills and monotonous exercises)
- In order to facilitate recovery of cognitive functions and to make rehabilitation fun, use video or board games that present some cognitive challenges appropriate to the child's strengths and weaknesses
- Focus, when appropriate, on academic skills and ways of integrating Cognitive Rehabilitation plans with school and classroom functioning

- Educate the child's peers and friends about the injury and its potential effects on behavior and cognition
- Encourage age-appropriate social and recreational activities, even if still in the hospital
- Compensatory strategies and other Cognitive Rehabilitation activities will be necessary for children who exhibit impairments with Attention, Memory, Perceptual Functioning, Problem Solving, motor coordination, and academic skills such as reading, math, and written expression
- Monitor behavioral dyscontrol and treat with Behavior Management techniques as appropriate
- Consider Social Skills Training or social skills groups for the child as necessary
- Encourage parents to maintain expectations for the child for appropriate behavior at home and in the community and to be consistent with their disciplining practices (parents tend to relax their parental control and discipline for the injured child upon return home, which in time can exacerbate behavioral problems)
- Changes in the child's educational plan may need to be made in order for the child to return to school (see School Placement/Considerations and Individualized Educational Program)

Mild TBI in Children

- Some controversy exists about the effects of mild TBI in children (see also Mild Traumatic Brain Injury)
- Although temporary changes in cognition and behavior have been reported in mild TBI, group studies have not consistently revealed long-term or persistent deficits
- Possible cognitive problems during the acute recovery period may include:
  - Memory
  - Motor speed
  - Reaction time
- Possible behavioral problems during the acute recovery period may include:
  - Irritability

    - "Clinging" behavior (increased dependence, helplessness, age regression)
    - Sleep disturbance
    - Headache
- Premorbid personality and family functioning may play an important role in long-term adaptive functioning
    - A child's injury may exacerbate family dysfunction
    - The child may develop long-term behavior problems due to decreased expectations for appropriate behavior
- Slight modifications with school may be necessary temporarily
    - Slight decrease in workload
    - Extra time for assignments

Fletcher, J. M., Ewing-Cobbs, L., Miner, M. E., Levin, H. S., & Eisenberg, H. M. (1990). Behavioral changes after closed head injury in children. *Journal of Consulting and Clinical Psychology, 58*, 93–98.

Jaffe, K. M., Fay, G. C., Polissar, N. L., et al. (1993). Severity of pediatric traumatic brain injury and neurobehavioral recovery at one year—A cohort study. *Archives of Physical Medicine and Rehabilitation, 74*, 587–595.

Michaud, L. J., Rivara, F. P., Jaffe, K. M., Fay, G., & Dailey, J. L. (1993). Traumatic brain injury as a risk factor for behavioral disorders in children. *Archives of Physical Medicine and Rehabilitation, 74*, 368–375.

Petrocelli, R. W., Guilmette, T. J., & McNamara, M. E. (1994). *Traumatic brain injury: Evaluation and litigation*. Charlottesville, VA: The Michie Company.

Trigeminal Nerve. Cranial Nerve V; its major functions are to convey sensation from the face and to innervate the muscles that protrude and close the jaw necessary for chewing; the three sensory divisions of the Trigeminal Nerve include the forehead (and cornea), cheek, and jaw; trigeminal neuralgia (tic douloureux), which can be caused by irritation to the nerve results in severe facial pain; the motor portion of this nerve originates in the Pons but the sensory portion extends from the Midbrain through the Medulla.

Trochlear Nerve. Cranial Nerve IV; one of the group of Cranial Nerves (with III and VI) that work together to move the eyes in unison (i.e., conjugate gaze); the Trochlear Nerve specifically controls the eye muscles for downward movement when the eye is turned inward; the Trochlear Nerve originates in the Midbrain.

Tumor (Brain). A growth of abnormal tissue in the brain that may be benign (noncancerous) or malignant (cancerous).

- Brain tumors typically develop insidiously in young and middle-aged adults and may present with a wide range of initial symptoms such as headache, Seizures, Depression, cognitive problems, or alterations in Personality (depending on the site of the tumor)
- Brain tumors may be relatively encapsulated or spread diffusely throughout adjacent brain tissue
- Most primary brain tumors arise from the connective tissue of the central nervous system, called glial cells (which include astrocytes and oligodendrocytes), and are named after their original cell line
- Gliomas (tumors that arise from glial cells) consist of a group of tumors called Astrocytomas and Glioblastomas, the latter being highly malignant and infiltrating
- Oligodendrogliomas are also a form of Gliomas but are somewhat rare and slow growing
- Treatment of brain tumors may include surgery, radiation therapy, and/or chemotherapy
- Cognitive Rehabilitation for patients with brain tumors may be necessary due to the direct effect of the tumor itself upon important brain structures as well as the effect of the surgery

Kaufman, D. M. (1995). *Clinical neurology for psychiatrists.* Philadelphia, PA: W. B. Saunders Company.

Utilization Behavior. An instrumentally correct but highly exaggerated response to environmental cues and objects; for example, patients may grab objects in their environment (pens, pencils, eating utensils, etc.) and use them even though they have no need or purpose in doing so; this occurs most frequently with lesions to the Frontal Lobes; see also Stimulus Bound.

Vagus Nerve. Cranial Nerve X; one of the Bulbar Nerves that arise from the Brain Stem and controls swallowing, phonation, and movement of the uvula and the soft palate; it also supplies sensation to the mucosa of the pharynx, soft palate, tonsils, and viscera of the thorax and abdomen.

Vasospasm. Defined as the narrowing of arteries in the Circle of Willis that occurs in approximately 50% of patients who survive a Subarachnoid Hemorrhage (SAH); the vasospasms result in impaired cerebral profusion or blood flow which may cause delayed Ischemia by impairing distal blood flow and increasing the potential for rebleeding of Aneurysms; they can occur between 3–12 days post-SAH but are most common in days 4–8; there is no known cause.

Bell, T. E., LaGrange, K. M., Maier, C. M., & Steinberg, G. K. (1992). Transcranial doppler: Correlation of blood velocity measurement with clinical status in subarachnoid hemorrhage. *Journal of Neuroscience Nursing, 24,* 215–219.

Ventricles. Pouches or spaces within the brain that contain Cerebrospinal Fluid (CSF); the two largest ventricles are the lateral ventricles which are located within each of the cerebral hemispheres, running front to back and curving around the Temporal Lobes; two smaller ventricles, the third and fourth ventricles, are located in the Brain Stem; CSF is produced by and travels through all the ventricles although the preponderance of CSF is produced in the lateral ventricles; if the ventricles enlarge, then additional pressure can be placed on other brain structures and result in mental status changes; see also Hydrocephalus, Shunt, and Normal Pressure Hydrocephalus.

Vertebral Artery. Two large arteries that converge at the Brain Stem to form the Basilar Artery which then enters the Circle of Willis and provides the arterial blood supply for Posterior brain structures; see Cerebral Circulation.

Vertigo. A sensation that one is spinning or that the environment is itself spinning; the most common causes are viral, Ischemia, or traumatic damage to the vestibular division of the Acoustic Nerve.

Viral Encephalopathy. A global and nonspecific term for brain damage that occurs due to viral infections; see Herpes Simplex Encephalitis.

Visual Analogue Mood Scale. A self-report measure of subjective distress used with neurologic patients who are unable to communicate verbally due to Aphasia following Cerebrovasular Accidents; the patient is shown a simple cartoon "happy face" at the top of a page and a corresponding "sad face" at the bottom separated by a 100 mm vertical line and then asked to place a mark on the line at the point that represents his or her degree of sadness.

Stern, R. A., & Bachman, D. L. (1991). Depressive symptoms following stroke. *American Journal of Psychiatry, 148*, 351-356.

Stern, R. A., Rosenbaum, J., White, R. F., & Morey, C. E. (1991). Clinical validation of a visual analogue dysphoria scale of neurologic patients. *Journal of Clinical and Experimental Neuropsychology, 13*, 106.

Visual Spatial Ability. See Perceptual Functioning.

Visual Field Cut. An area of blindness within the visual fields caused by a disruption in the optic tracts from the eyes to the Occipital Lobes; it is much more easily compensated for than visual Neglect because it is not a disorder of spatial Attention; field cuts can co-occur with Neglects; see also Hemianopsia.

Vocational Rehabilitation. The use of rehabilitation principles to assist persons to return to work on either a part-time or full-time basis following a disabling condition or disorder.

- In Traumatic Brain Injury, approximately 20% to 40% of patients are able to return to competitive employment (some persons with TBI are able to return to part-time or less competitive employment)
- For younger adults, working or being productive (if even in a limited capacity) is very important for self-esteem and to promote positive feelings of self-worth

- The ability to return to work may occur very late in the recovery process (e.g., greater than 2–4 years postinjury)

Predicting Employment Following Brain Injury

- Multiple variables are important in whether persons with TBI are able to return to work
- Preinjury variables
  - Age (>60 years of age is associated with poor rates of returning to work)
  - Work history (e.g., steady work history, employed at time of injury)
  - Type of job at the time of injury and skills necessary to fulfill job requirements sucessfully
- Injury variables
  - Longer lengths of Coma are related to poorer vocational outcome
  - Longer lengths of Posttraumatic Amnesia (PTA) are related to poorer vocational outcome (one study has revealed that with greater than 33 days of PTA, none of 36 patients regained prior employment status)
  - The greater the severity of neurologic damage, the less likely the patient will be capable of returning to work
- Postinjury variables
  - Financial incentives
  - Availability of work
  - Availability of rehabilitation programs
  - ADL status
- Cognitive/psychosocial impairments that impede returning to work
  - Executive Functions
  - Anosmia
  - Mental Speed
  - Fatigability
  - Awareness of deficits
  - Depression, irritability, paranoia
  - Schwab (1993) reported that the seven most important variables in predicting the work status of Vietnam veterans 15 years after penetrating head injury included Sei-

zures, paresis, Visual Field Cuts, verbal and visual Memory loss, psychological/Adjustment problems, and violent behavior

Suggestions for Vocational Rehabilitation

- It is easier to train persons for specific jobs rather than for the world of work in general
- Formal vocational rehabilitation treatment typically begins when the major cognitive and physical deficits have stabilized
- Identify how work is done at the patient's place of employment (conduct work site evaluation or functional analysis if possible)
  - Amount of supervision
  - Amount of interpersonal interaction with co-workers or with the public
  - Amount of variability and predictability in a work day
  - Time demands
- Vocational assessment
  - Assess specific job-related skills (e.g., motor speed and coordination for an assembly position or reading comprehension for a job that requires extensive reading)
  - Conduct neuropsychological assessment
  - Conduct occupational, physical, and speech-language therapy evaluations as necessary
  - Conduct simulated job appraisal (i.e., if possible, test job-specific skills in a simulated work environment)
  - Interview family members to assess interpersonal and behavioral functioning
- Assess Adjustment to injury and disability
  - Evaluate expectations for returning to work
  - The goal for the patient is to be PRODUCTIVE (doing something is better than doing nothing, even if the something isn't as good or isn't just like it was before the injury)
  - Motivation and commitment to work are crucial
  - Psychotherapy or counseling may be necessary
- Refine insight and Awareness about the patients' strengths and weaknesses as they pertain to the world of work

- Teach specific skills necessary for a specific type of work (i.e., domain specific skills)
- Try to capitalize on previously learned skills, knowledge, or interests
- Assess and treat work-related social behaviors (e.g. timeliness, ability to receive criticism, relationships with co-workers and supervisors, etc.)
- Use Behavior Management and/or Social Skills Training for problematic interpersonal behaviors
- Break down tasks into small steps that can be mastered
- Make therapy as much like the work setting as possible
- Rely on external cues and compensatory aids as necessary (e.g., daily checklists, visual aids, written reminders); see Memory and Memory Log
- Use job coaches as necessary
- Volunteer or part-time work are good ways to try out skills or new techniques
- Provide as much on-site help as the patient requires
- Treat substance abuse if present (see Alcohol Effects)
- Educate employers and co-workers

Guilmette, T. J., & Kastner, M. P. (1996). The prediction of vocational functioning from neuropsychological data. In R. Sbordone & C. Long (Eds.), *Ecological validity of neuropsychological testing* (pp. 387–412). Delray Beach, FL: GR Press/St. Lucie Press.

Schwab, K., Grafman, J., Salazar, A. M., & Kraft, J. (1993). Residual impairments and work status 15 years after penetrating head injury: Report from the Vietnam Head Injury Study. *Neurology, 43*, 95–103.

Vocabulary. One of the subtests of the Wechsler Adult Intelligence Scale—Revised and the Wechsler Intelligence Scale for Children—III which assesses word knowledge or expressive vocabulary; it is affected by level of education and socioeconomic background; vocabulary can also provide an estimate of premorbid verbal functioning in patients who do not have Aphasia or who do not have extensive left hemisphere damage.

Wechsler Adult Intelligence Scale—Revised (WAIS-R). The most popular and best standardized, individually administered Intelligence Test for persons ages 16–74 (although additional norms have been published which extend the upper age for which the WAIS-R can be used); it can be differentially affected by neurologic disorders, including TBI; it is composed of 11 subtests (Information, Digit Span, Vocabulary, Arithmetic, Comprehension, Similarities, Picture Completion, Picture Arrangement, Block Design, Object Assembly, and Digit Symbol) which are based on a mean of 10 and a standard deviation of 3 (see Test Scores); the WAIS-R yields three IQ scores (Verbal, Performance, and Full Scale).

Wechsler, D. (1981). *WAIS-R manual.* New York, NY: The Psychological Corporation.

Wechsler Intelligence Scale for Children—III (WISC-III). The most popular and best standardized, individually administered Intelligence Test for children ages 6–16 years, 11 months; it can be differentially affected by neurologic disorders, including TBI (see Traumatic Brain Injury-Pediatric); the WISC-III is composed of the following subtests: Information, Similarities, Arithmetic, Vocabulary, Comprehension, Digit Span, Picture Completion, Coding, Picture Arrangement, Block Design, Object Assembly, Symbol Search, and Mazes; the subtest scores are reported with a mean of 10 and a standard deviation of 3 (see Test Scores); the WISC-III yields three global IQ scores (Verbal, Performance, and Full Scale).

Wechsler, D. (1991). *WISC-III manual.* New York, NY: The Psychological Corporation.

Wechsler Memory Scale—Revised (WMS-R). One of the most commonly used, standardized batteries for the assessment of Memory for persons ages 16–74 (although additional norms have been published that extend the upper age with which the WMS-R can be used); the WMS-R is composed of several subtests and yields global indices for verbal Memory, visual Memory, general Memory, Attention/Concentration, and delayed recall; the WMS-R is sensitive to most Memory disorders of varying etiologies.

Wechsler, D. (1987). *WMS-R manual.* New York, NY: The Psychological Corporation.

Western Neuro Sensory Stimulation Profile. A 33-item test that assesses cognitive/communicative functions in noncomatose, low functioning patients; six major areas of functioning are assessed, including Arousal/Attention, auditory comprehension, visual comprehension, visual tracking, object manipulation, and expressive communication.

Ansell, B. J. (1993). Slow-to-recover patients: Improvement to rehabilitation readiness. *Journal of Head Trauma Rehabilitation, 8, 88–98.*

Ansell, B., Keenan, J., & de la Rocha, O. (1989). *Western Neuro Sensory Stimulation Profile.* Tustin, CA: Western Neuro Care Center.

White Matter. The densely packed Axons that transmit neural information from points within a cerebral hemisphere, between cerebral hemispheres (see Corpus Callosum), or between the Cortex and lower brain structures; white matter lesions occur most commonly from trauma to the brain (see Diffuse Axonal Injury), vascular disorders, and demyelinating disorders such as Multiple Sclerosis, and tend to result in attentional problems and decreased Mental Speed; lesions to the white matter can also result in Dementia and Depression.

Wide Range Achievement Test—3 (WRAT-3). A standardized and individually administered measure of single word reading, spelling, and written arithmetic; this Achievement Test can be sensitive to Learning Disabilities and academic functioning; the reading subtest can help provide an estimate of premorbid intellectual functioning in persons of normal intelligence and without a history of learning problems.

Wilkinson, G. S. (1993). *The Wide Range Achievement Test Administration Manual.* Wilmington, DE: Wide Range, Inc.

Wisconsin Card Sorting Test (WCST). A measure of Abstract and Conceptual Thinking that requires the person to shift Problem Solving strategies in response to changing environmental contingencies by sorting a deck of response cards according to their characteristics based on examiner feedback of whether the patient's sorting strategy is correct or incorrect; the WCS appears sensitive to difficulties with Executive Functioning, although not to Frontal Lobe damage specifically; it is administered with few instructions and so may also provide some measure of frustration tolerance and ability to manage ambiguity.

Heaton, R. K. et al. (1993). *Wisconsin Card Sorting Test Manual: Revised and expanded.* Odessa, FL: Psychological Assessment Resources.

About the Author

Thomas J. Guilmette, Ph.D., ABPP is Director of Neuropsychology at Rhode Island Hospital and the Southern New England Rehbilitation Center at the St. Joseph Hospital for Specialty Care, both in Providence, Rhode Island. He is also a Clinical Assistant Professor at Brown University Medical School and serves as a consultant to the Southeastern Rehabilitation Center at Charlton Memorial Hospital in Fall River, Massachusetts.

Dr. Guilmette received his bachelor's degree in Psychology from Providence College and his doctorate in Counseling Psychology from the University of Missouri. He completed a two-year postdoctoral fellowship in adult and pediatric neuropsychology at Brown University and is board certified in clinical neuropsychology by the American Academy of Clinical Neuropsychology and the American Board of Professional Psychology. Dr. Guilmette has worked in brain injury rehbilitation for over 10 years and has published more than 30 professional papers in the field of neuropsychology and related areas.